Cesarean Birth

Cesarean Birth

A COUPLE'S GUIDE FOR DECISION AND PREPARATION

Revised Edition

Kathleen Mitchell
Marty Nason, R.N.

Beaufort Books ▪ Publishers

New York

Library of Congress Cataloging in Publication Data

Mitchell, Kathleen.
    Cesarean birth.

    Rev. ed. of: Cesarean childbirth, ©1981.
    Bibliography: p.
    Includes index.
    1. Cesarean section.   I. Nason, Marty.   II. Mitchell, Kathleen. Cesarean childbirth.
III. Title.
[DNLM: 1. Cesarean Section—popular works. WQ 150 M6814]
[RG761.M57 1985] 618.8′6 84-28266
ISBN 0-8253-0275-7 (pbk.)

Published in the United States by Beaufort Books Publishers, New York.

Designer: Libra Graphics, Inc.

Printed in the U.S.A.   First Beaufort Edition

10 9 8 7 6 5 4 3 2 1

Dedication

We dedicate this book to
EVERY EXPECTANT COUPLE

Acknowledgments

We would like to express our appreciation to those who supported and encouraged us as we worked to write this book. Especially Mitch and Jim.

Many cesarean couples shared their experiences and feelings with us, especially Bobbin and Steve Yarbrough, Leslie and Harry Leff, and Barbara Kalmen.

Many doctors were most generous with their time, especially Jack Klausen, Jerome Ratzen, Cheriyn Sheets, and Gary Oaks.

We are grateful to Jack and Barbara Bulko, who pictorially shared with us the birth of their son, Aran Edward.

Other family members and friends contributed their assistance in various ways: Suzanne, Julie, Rob, Andrea, Sarah, Inez and William Beye, Ethyl Blake. And, Elisabeth Bing, R.P.T., childbirth author and educator, gave us her expert assistance.

A very special thanks to Bob Mitchell for generously giving his time for editorial assistance, and without whose help this book would not have been written.

Contents

Introduction

by David Horowitz

I have never dealt with an issue closer to my heart or perhaps more controversial than the rights of cesarean parents.

Shortly after the birth of my daughter, I had the opportunity to discuss my cesarean birth experience on national television. On that program, I said that the cesarean birth came as a total surprise for my wife Suzanne and me. The obstetrician told us that our baby was too big to be born through the birth canal.

My wife and I had taken the Lamaze childbirth course in anticipation of a joyful, shared birth experience. When an emergency surgical birth became necessary, there was, at that point, no way to adjust our preparations to share it. We were disappointed, because I was to have helped in the vaginal delivery, but the doctor wanted me to leave the operating room during the cesarean. I felt there was no reason for me to be excluded. I wanted to share the birth experience and lend support to my wife, who needed all the reinforcement and support she could get.

The doctor emphatically refused to let me remain in the operating room. However, after some discussion he did consent to my re-

David Horowitz is a cesarean father. He is NBC's Consumer Reporting Specialist and winner of three Emmy Awards. He appears frequently on many national talk shows and is seen regularly on NBC television programs. Horowitz's daily radio feature "Fight Back!" is aired on over 250 stations on the NBC radio network. He is the creator, host, and executive producer of the syndicated television production "Fight Back! With David Horowitz." Horowitz is the author of Fight Back! And Don't Get Ripped Off *(Harper & Row, 1979).*

turning when the surgery was completed and the baby was born. We had agreed earlier that I would be allowed to cut the baby's umbilical cord and give the baby its first bath. The doctor kept his end of the bargain. I told him, however, that I felt no husband should be excluded from sharing this experience with his wife; he should be at her side if he wants to be. Prospective parents should be able to take a cesarean childbirth class, to teach them what will happen if a cesarean is required. I also thought doctors should advise expectant couples that surprise cesareans are always possible. We found that traditional natural childbirth classes do not spend enough time discussing cesarean births.

The public response to hearing my experience was overwhelming. I received thousands of letters from all over the country. I had definitely struck a nerve. This did not surprise me, considering the intensity of Suzanne's and my own feelings on the subject of cesarean birth. What did surprise me was the great number of people affected —approximately one out of every five births is by cesarean. That statistic surprises almost everyone!

Those of you who watch my syndicated "Fight Back!" program are familiar with the "Fight Back! Fact File." The file cabinet contains the mail we receive from our viewers describing rip-off incidents and consumers' complaints of injustice perpetrated by various companies and institutions across the country. Let me share with you some excerpts from the letters I received from cesarean parents regarding how they felt about their cesarean experience.

- "It did me so much good to hear you talk about your frustration with your cesarean. I just had a cesarean, too. I can't seem to be able to communicate my feelings of frustrations to anyone, including my husband and my doctor. You weren't happy with your experience, either. I think people will listen to you. I sure hope you can change things for us cesarean parents. Good Luck."

- "I felt like a freak when my parents and in-laws talked about my 'abnormal' delivery."

- "My cesarean was so frightening to me that if it wasn't for my religious beliefs I would never have another baby."

- "I felt like my baby was deprived of something. I felt deprived."

- "I keep telling myself that I just gave birth to a baby. I don't feel like I did."

- "My husband and I were so disappointed. We were doing so well in our Lamaze class. We had such high expectations."

- "We felt bitter that we were not allowed to participate in the birth of our son. That miracle moment was denied us, and nothing on earth can bring that moment back to us. Maybe it shouldn't matter so much, but I can't have any more children."

- "I was absolutely livid that my doctor had not warned us that a cesarean is always a possibility and we should prepare for that possibility."

I also received dozens of letters from cesarean support groups notifying me of their existence and explaining their objectives and goals. I received letters from concerned cesarean childbirth instructors telling me of their programs and the various locations of these classes. I was pleased to learn that these groups existed, but the basic questions still remained: "Why don't more people know about these classes and organizations? Why isn't the medical community promoting these groups and cooperating with them to improve the cesarean experience? How many people, such as myself, find out about them after the fact?"

Admittedly, not all cesarean experiences are emotionally distressing. Many cesarean parents have positive experiences. Certainly most doctors are skilled in performing successful surgery. *But this is not the issue.* The outrage stems from the insensitivity of so much of the medical community to the *feelings* of the cesarean mother and father.

It was gratifying to hear from many people who had the good fortune to have been told about, and to attend, a cesarean childbirth class in order to hear what such a birth can be like when one is prepared and permitted to participate. Unfortunately, my mail was largely from dissatisfied parents looking for a better way.

As a consumer reporting specialist with a reputation built on helping others to "Fight Back!" as well as being a cesarean father, I am in a unique position to advise cesarean parents of their rights and to encourage them to strive for better ways of improving the total cesarean experience. As you know, I tell millions of television viewers each week to fight back and not get ripped off. What do I mean when I say that? I don't expect angry, pregnant women to rush to their obstetrician's office and beat their doctors up with this book. Your weapons are being aware, being informed, making your wishes known, and being ready to go to bat for your beliefs in a nice, dignified way. I call it "righteous indignation." Any doctor must respect that. The relationship between the obstetrician and the patient should be harmonious. It should be a partnership between the expectant couple, who are seeking a safe and meaningful cesarean birth experience, and the doctor, who provides service with professional knowledge, expertise, and empathy.

Doctors and hospital staff exist to serve you. Often, as patients, we lose sight of this fact. We don't want to bother the nurses, we often don't dare ask the doctors any questions because we feel intimidated. When you feel this way, just ask yourself, "Whose body and whose baby are in question, and who is paying the bill?" Don't suffer or worry in silence.

You should also remember that, in order for the doctors and nurses to help, you must make your wishes known. You must know your rights.

You have a right to know what is happening at all times, and why.

You have a right to know what anesthesia you will be receiving and what its effects are. You have a right to meet with your anesthesiologist before going to the hospital, or at the hospital before the surgery, to discuss the various anesthetics, and to state a preference, if you have one. Of course, to have an educated preference you must be informed.

You have the right to request tests to determine fetal maturity. You have a right to an explanation of the tests and the advantages and disadvantages associated with each.

You have the right to express a preference for hospital procedures, such as scheduling the hour for the cesarean surgery, having your husband present for the delivery (if you are prepared and this is your desire), rooming-in privileges, sibling visitation rights, and the like.

You have a right to know what drugs have been prescribed for you for pain medication and so on. You have a right to know how they will affect you. You have the right to accept or reject such medication.

You have the right to see your baby in the operating room and also for a time in the recovery room if you both are healthy.

You have the right to breastfeed your baby.

Now I must tell you that you have the right, legally, to refuse a cesarean by not signing the consent form. You would probably have to sign a waiver absolving the hospital from problems resulting from a difficult and dangerous vaginal birth. I *don't recommend that you do this,* but you should be aware that it is your right to do so. In general, keep in mind that it is your right to be treated with consideration and respect.

If you are treated badly or ignored while you are in the hospital, you have the right and even the duty to fight back. It's pretty hard to do much when you are lying helpless and uncomfortable in a hospital bed with stitches in your tummy and possibly an IV needle in your arm. So enlist help from your husband, parents, and friends. You may seek help from your doctor, the head nurse, the pediatrician, or the hospital administrator. When you get back home, write letters to the hospital and the doctors.

In the past, women haven't known much about cesarean delivery, so they have given full control over all decisions, large or small, to the doctors. Times are changing. Parents today are not always willing to passively accept the rigid and routine procedure established for all women alike without consideration for individual concerns. Women are better informed, more inquisitive, and in search of better answers. They want more than to have a healthy baby and to come through surgery unharmed. They want a meaningful and joyful childbirth experience.

Cesarean parents are now just beginning to see changes in obstetric care resulting from "consumer power." They can look back to the success of the Lamaze method of childbirth in our country as one source of the changes now affecting them. When this method of childbirth was introduced in the United States, women insisted on having the option to deliver their babies in this manner. Consumer pressure was great, and eventually the hospitals accommodated them. Doctors and hospitals must respond to what their patients want in order to avoid losing their customers.

In this country, the women's movement and the consumer movement have grown up together; books such as this one are a natural outgrowth of these movements. This book is a consumer guide to the cesarean birth experience. It challenges many traditional policies and practices regarding cesarean delivery and advises the reader of the rights and options of cesarean parents. I recommend this book for all prospective parents. It is objective and easy to read. It deals with controversial issues with understanding and candor. And it gives parents the information and awareness that is necessary in order to *Fight Back!*

Cesarean Delivery: Background

CHAPTER ONE

It Could Happen to You

I am a cesarean mother. Like most women, I wanted a vaginal birth; in fact, I had never seriously contemplated the possibility of a cesarean. I found out too late, like so many others, that it is often not possible or not advisable to deliver vaginally. Did you know that at least one birth out of every five will be by cesarean this year? For many women involved, the delivery will be repeat surgery. For others, the cesarean will be unexpected. Unfortunately, in most first cesareans the doctor is not able to determine that a cesarean is required until the woman is well into labor.

Among those most disappointed and frustrated by a cesarean birth are couples who went through Lamaze, or a similar childbirth preparation class, anticipating a joyous and shared birth only to discover at the last minute a cesarean would have to be performed. The father who has been trained only for natural childbirth now has nothing to do but pace the floor, disappointed, angry, and frightened for his wife and baby. He feels useless, superfluous, and bewildered. He may even feel guilty. All the training, planning, and anticipation was for nothing. The situation is out of the frightened couple's control. The laboring mother is wheeled away from her helpmate to the operating room. She is alarmed for her baby and for herself. *Does this trauma have to be?*

This is the question that I, a three-time cesarean mother and co-author of this book, asked myself after my first cesarean. The wonderful experience in childbirth that my husband Bob and I had planned turned into a nightmarish emergency cesarean. Physically, I made a full recovery from surgery. I had only the scar to remind me. Emotionally, I was left with unseen scars. I felt a bitter conviction that what I had suffered psychologically was not necessary. I was amazed that the doctors who were so technically skilled and successful in performing the surgery itself totally ignored the human aspects of childbirth. I told myself I should just be happy that I had a healthy baby. I tried to push the whole episode out of my mind. Actually, my mental defenses were already at work, because I had blocked most of it out. However, the nightmare returned. Two weeks after surgery, just as I began to doze off for a nap, I relived the surgery. I could hear the doctors talking to each other. The memories flooded in as though a dam in my head had broken. I began to tremble and cry. I tried to push the whole episode out of my mind, but I couldn't. I felt angry and betrayed.

When I went for my postnatal checkup, I told my doctor how I felt. I told him that mothers should be warned by their obstetricians that a cesarean delivery is always a possibility for anyone and that expectant mothers should receive some preparation so that in the event of a cesarean they wouldn't be shocked and afraid. I told him what had gone through my head at the time: "I didn't know what was happening. I just knew that something had gone wrong and I was going to have a cesarean. I thought maybe my baby was going to die or be abnormal. I thought maybe I was going to die, too." I told him there was no reason I should have suffered from these torturing thoughts. I could accept my physical pain—I understood that. But to have suffered emotionally at the same time was inexcusable, when a few words of explanation and encouragement would have been so simple, and would have avoided so much trauma.

My doctor was amazed. He had never considered the things I was telling him in that light. "I'm truly sorry," he said. "I didn't know." I went away hoping that the next patient to walk into his office, and every patient from then on, would benefit from what I was able to convey to him that day.

What happened to me is very typical. Medical schools teach young men and women modern technical expertise. Too often, however, they neglect the emotional and the psychological aspects of childbirth, including maternal-infant bonding, the importance of the father's participation in the delivery, nutrition, and the art of breast-feeding. If doctors were more aware of these areas, perhaps this book would not need to be written! But until a holistic approach to prenatal care becomes routine, couples must take it on themselves to be prepared for cesarean birth. Otherwise, the surprise cesarean can be a cruel blow to you, the expectant couple. The cesarean is not a low-risk procedure in a psychological sense. Cesarean couples sometimes suffer severe trauma from being thrust into a cesarean situation unprepared and ill informed.

I wanted to have another baby but I was afraid to go through another cesarean. At that point in time having a vaginal birth after a cesarean would not have been even considered, so that was not even an option for me. Finally I did decide to get pregnant again. I was wondering, as you may be, "What is a repeat, planned cesarean like?" On the positive side, there is no labor to go through. Generally, you are awake until the baby is born. You are, of course, numb from your breasts to your toes. Depending on the mother's preference, or the doctor's, the mother is sometimes put to sleep for the entire procedure. Either way, it is a lonely, unfulfilling way to give birth.

In my second, planned cesarean birth, I remember how much I hated saying goodbye to Bob and being wheeled to the operating room. I was very nervous the entire time. No one ever looked at me or said anything to me. I felt invisible. More accurately, I felt not like a whole woman but like a bulging abdomen ready to be opened and relieved of its contents. The atmosphere was cold and clinical. When the baby was finally born, someone said, "You have a baby girl." I strained to see, but my wrists were strapped. I saw her back as someone lifted her by the feet, and then I was put to sleep. I didn't see her again for at least a day. Again I felt strongly that I had missed out on what could have been a special time for me. I felt sad that cesarean parents were missing the joys and benefits that other couples enjoyed.

The third time I became pregnant, I knew it was to be my last baby, and I resolved that somehow this was going to be a better experience. I had no idea then just how different it was going to be! It was my great good fortune to find a doctor who was sensitive to the emotional aspects of childbirth. He had long ago pioneered and promoted the Lamaze method in our area. We discussed my previous deliveries and my unhappiness with the cesarean procedure. He had independently arrived at my same conclusion: Women needed to be prepared for cesareans. "Furthermore," he said, "I believe the cesarean delivery can and should be a warm, human, and possibly shared experience." He explained that he had just instituted a cesarean childbirth class under the direction of Marty Nason, a nurse and childbirth educator, who eventually became the co-author of this book on prepared cesarean childbirth.

My doctor said, "If Bob wishes, he may also take the class and prepare to be with you for the birth. He will not observe the surgery; his role would be to sit at your head where he can talk to you, hold your hand, lend you support, and share the joy of the birth with you.'' I was overwhelmed. I thought I might like to have Bob with me. However, I wasn't at all sure that *he* would want to be in the surgical suite, even when the doctor explained that Bob would not see the surgery but would just sit at my head, hold my hand, and lend support. He would get to hold the baby right after its birth and would bring the baby to me to see. I was grateful for the doctor's concern in trying to make the cesarean experience warm and human, even though it was surgery, but I was going to have to think about having Bob in the operating room with me!

For the next couple of weeks, Bob and I thought about and discussed the pros and cons of his sharing the birth experience with me. We both had some reservations to overcome. I was secretly afraid that Bob might find such an experience a turn-off and that it might affect the way he felt about me and the baby. What if he got sick? How would that affect the doctors? Surgery is serious business. Would our family approve? Would our friends think we were silly to want to share in a cesarean birth? Would Bob tell his colleagues at work? Would they kid him about it?

Bob was also worried he might react negatively to being with me during surgery and, instead of helping me, might make matters worse. He wasn't sure what would be expected of him. Would he let me down or somehow make a fool of himself?

In the final analysis, our desire to be together far outweighed all our fears. This was to be our last baby, and we wanted to savor every joy. We also wanted to know for ourselves if cesarean parents could share the same joys as parents who share vaginal delivery.

Marty Nason prepared us for every aspect of the cesarean experience. We learned what to expect every step of the way. She helped us resolve negative feelings about the cesarean delivery held over from our past experiences. We talked with the anesthesiologist. We toured the maternity ward. We saw the surgical suite. Bob got to see the green surgical gown he would be wearing. I was planning to breast-feed my baby for the first time and was feeling good about the decision. When the big day arrived, it turned out to be a totally different childbirth experience from anything I had experienced in the past.

Once surgery was underway and Bob was at my side, I wasn't frightened at all. I was excited. It only took about five minutes for the baby to be born, and it seemed shorter than that to me. The anesthesiologist spoke to Bob and me several times to tell us that I was doing well and that the surgery was progressing well. When the baby was about to be born, the anesthesiologist said to Bob, "Stand up if you want, your baby is being born." Bob squeezed my hand and stood up. I will never forget his expression of awe and delight. As soon as the baby had been briefly examined, she was brought to us to see. Bob held her. I reached out and touched her little foot, then her tiny fingers. I felt a pleasure and pride in being a woman and a mother that I had never experienced in quite the same way before. I didn't feel invisible. I had no memories to block out. I had memories to cherish: how my baby looked when she first came into the world, Bob's happiness, my own good feelings about myself, and my relationship with my husband and my newborn.

Bob, whose prior experience with childbirth had been pacing the floor in the waiting room, was elated. He was thrilled to see his daughter born—to hold her close to him as she gleaned her first impressions of the world. It was a special moment for us, one that helped bond us to our child.

Having experienced three completely different emotional reactions to cesarean childbirth, I felt I was in a unique position to help other couples achieve a satisfying cesarean birth experience. But with the demands of a new baby I let a year lapse before I made a date to talk to Marty, who was involved in many different areas of cesarean childbirth education, such as teaching classes, working with the local cesarean support group, giving seminars, and doing work on public relations. Her work with cesarean couples made her realize the enormity of the problems such parents were facing. These problems were particularly severe for unprepared couples who experienced a surprise cesarean.

Marty explained, "When I first began working with cesarean parents and heard their accounts of fear, rage, disappointment, and guilt at the unexpected turn of events surrounding the childbirth, I had a difficult time relating to the intensity of their feelings. But as I kept hearing the same stories over, and over, and over, I became convinced of the magnitude of the problem. In order to prepare them for a positive experience, I attended dozens of actual births and witnessed the profound difference it made when the couples were prepared and shared the birth experience. I began devoting a large portion of class time to helping cesarean couples resolve the negative emotions they harbored."

Two things became clear to us. First, parents, prospective parents, doctors, hospitals, and childbirth instructors must all work together to make the cesarean delivery a better total experience than it has been in the past. Second, couples must take the responsibility for preparing themselves for a cesarean childbirth and for taking advantage of the various birth options now available.

Marty and I decided to write a guide on prepared cesarean childbirth that could be used as a textbook in cesarean childbirth classes and, more importantly, could be made available to every expectant couple, whether anticipating a cesarean or vaginal delivery. With a cesarean rate of 20 to 25 percent, *every* expectant parent must be prepared for the possibility of a surgical delivery.

Our experience has shown that several factors have a tremendous impact on the couple's perception of the cesarean experience. One factor is knowing what to expect. If fear of the unknown is replaced with understanding, couples enjoy a much better experience. Therefore, this book is a complete guide to understanding every aspect of cesarean birth, from the time your pregnancy is confirmed, through your hospital experience, and home again.

You will learn the reasons for certain tests and procedures, how they are performed, how they might feel, and how to best cope with them. We have provided you with information about options such as breast- versus bottle-feeding, going into labor versus picking the date for your cesarean, having a vaginal delivery after a cesarean, and being asleep versus being awake for the surgery.

We also examine the role of the father in the cesarean delivery, as one of the major options. Traditionally, the father has been excluded, so it is not surprising that he often doesn't know what his feelings are about sharing a cesarean. Although some hospitals do not accept the father's presence in the surgical suite, more and more enlightened hospitals are promoting or at least accepting the father's right to be there.

The latest option for cesarean mothers, an extremely significant one, is the possibility of a vaginal delivery after a cesarean (VBAC, pronounced "VEEBAC"). We attempt to provide all the current information on the subject. We answer such questions as, "Who is a candidate for a VBAC? What are the risks and issues surrounding a trial of labor?"

We realize that some options discussed in this book are not available in every hospital in this country. For the woman or couple who has a strong commitment to getting the kind of birth experience she wants, we have included an important chapter on how to go about achieving this goal within the medical and hospital "establishment."

You will also learn the answers to such questions as "Is the saying 'Once a cesarean, always a cesarean' true? What physical exercises and diet are beneficial for a woman anticipating a cesarean? What are the signs of labor? What happens in the hospital? Is pain medication for nursing mothers harmful to the baby? Can cesarean mothers breast-feed?"

Learning about cesarean procedures and options and examining the birth experiences and viewpoints set forth in this book by the participants, both nonprofessional and professional, will give you a more informed basis for deciding on the type of cesarean birth you want should a cesarean be required. We believe that couples should not just "survive" a cesarean but should be enriched by it as a meaningful event. You should have the most satisfying and joyful birth experience possible. We think you deserve the best!

CHAPTER TWO

The Changing Cesarean Experience

There is an air of excitement in the delivery room. A woman has just had a vaginal delivery and looks so happy. Her husband is with her and they are smiling at their new baby. This may sound like a typical scene, but something is different. The woman had her previous baby by cesarean.

At last some doctors and hospitals are beginning to assist cesarean mothers in attempting a trial of labor leading to vaginal deliveries in subsequent pregnancies. Vaginal birth after a cesarean (VBAC pronounced "veebac") is a long overdue, but very exciting break from the traditional practice of automatically delivering by cesarean any woman who had previously had a cesarean. This development reflects recent studies showing that 50 to 80 percent of women who have had cesareans can deliver vaginally in later pregnancies if they do not: (i) have recurring conditions that make a cesarean necessary, or (ii) have a classical scar (vertical) from the past cesarean.[1]

VBAC's could herald the end of the escalating cesarean rate. Unfortunately, very few doctors or hospitals have been willing to participate in VBAC's. Recent guidelines propounded by the American College of Obstetrics and Gynecology for performing this procedure should encourage its greater use. VBAC's will become a more common occurence as consumer pressure for this birthing alternative will undoubtedly increase.

Let's move to the operating room and see what changes have occurred there. Looking through the window we see that the woman on the operating table is smiling at the man in the green surgical cap and gown. The expression on her face and the way she is holding his hand indicate there is a loving intimacy between them. This may strike you as odd but there is a simple explanation. The man is dressed like the doctors but he is not one of them; he is the woman's husband.

Father-attended cesarean births are now common scenes in most hospitals and serve as an example of the changes in delivery procedures resulting from the consumer demand for a more humanistic approach to cesarean birth.

To get a good idea of the significance of current developments in cesarean delivery, let's back up for a moment and briefly scan the history of surgical birth.

Suppose you were asked, "Where did the name *cesarean section* originate?" You would probably reply, "From Julius Caesar. He was the first person we know of who was born by this method of cutting the mother's uterus to remove the baby, so the procedure was named after him." If you were on a quiz show, you would lose the point. The game host would pull out the white answer card and say, "I'm sorry; but that is the wrong answer. According to *Principles and Practice of Obstetrics*, 'The term probably is derived from the Latin, *partus caesareus*, from *caedere*, to cut. There is no evidence to show that Julius Caesar was thus delivered. Caesones (children delivered by section from their dead mothers) were known long before Caesar's time, and the operation was not performed on the living in Rome. Caesar's mother was alive at the time of his wars, as is proven by his letters to her.' "[1]

Early records trace the origins of cesarean delivery to the reign of the Roman king Numa Pompilius (715–672 B.C.), who decreed that the child be removed from the womb of any woman who died in the last stages of pregnancy. This royal law continued througout the reigns of the Caesars, when it acquired the name *lex caesarea*.[2]

Another early legend suggests that Buddha was delivered by cesarean (approximately 563 B.C.), and Brahma is also thought to have been born through the umbilicus. Apparently, the practice of cesarean delivery was known among the ancient Jews, because the Talmud prescribes laws concerning hygiene for survivors of the operation.[3]

Early in the sixteenth century, a Swiss swine gelder named Nufer presumably performed a successful operation on his own wife after attempts at a vaginal delivery had failed. Trautman of Wittenberg reported doing a cesarean delivery in 1610.[4] (The patient survived until the twenty-fifth postoperative day, longer than most women would live after the operation for the next two centuries.)

By 1878 the operation had been performed eighty times in the United States. The mortality rate was about 50 percent.[5]

The first successful cesarean section in the United States was performed in 1794, in a cabin near Staunton, Virginia, by Dr. Jesse Bennett on his own wife. After Mrs. Bennett, a young primagravida, had labored for three days without result, consultation was obtained with Dr. Alexander Humphreys, a physician of greater experience, who confirmed Dr. Bennett's suspicion of contracted pelvis and the impossibility of a natural delivery, and proposed a destructive operation on the baby as the only means of saving the mother's life. Having already despaired of her own chances, Mrs. Bennett begged that a cesarean section be done, for the sake of the child. This, however, Dr. Humphreys steadfastly refused, stating that he would not be the cause of his patient's death. Under the importunings of his suffering wife, Dr. Bennett therefore announced to his older colleague that he himself would perform the operation and, if fate ordained, would assume the full responsibility for her death.

An operating table was improvised with two wooden planks, supported on barrels. Without anesthesia, and while two Negro women held his wife, Dr. Bennett rapidly incised her abdomen and uterus and extracted the living infant. To protect her against a recurrence of this ordeal, should she survive, he then quickly removed his wife's ovaries, before closing her abdomen with linen thread. Both mother and child did indeed survive; but despite its successful outcome, Dr. Bennett never reported the case. When questioned years later concerning his reticence, Bennett replied, "No strange doctors would believe that the operation could be done in the Virginia backwoods and the mother live, and I'll be damn'd if I'd give them a chance to call me a liar."[6]

The modern cesarean era began in 1840 with the introduction of anesthesia, which made possible rapid development of improved surgical methods, because the speed of surgery was no longer the primary consideration.

Postoperative infection then became the major problem confronting surgeons. Mothers were surviving surgery but dying from postoperative infection. The importance of having everything surrounding the incision sterile was not understood. This breakthrough resulted in a sharp decline in the mortality rate.

In 1882 Max Sanger performed surgery that became the classical method on which today's procedures are based. He developed a technique to close the uterine incision with sutures while avoiding infection. The suturing technique reduced the hazard of hemorrhage and made removing the uterus unnecessary.[7]

THE INCREASING CESAREAN SECTION RATE

The twentieth century brought modern advances in medical technology such as aseptic surgical techniques, improvement in anesthetic methods, development of safe blood transfusions, and the discovery of antibiotics. These developments made surgical delivery a low risk operation, no longer resorted to only in life-threatening situations.

Improved medical control of maternal illnesses, such as diabetes, heart disease, and hypertension resulted in a lowered cesarean maternal mortality rate. Accordingly, this removed the reluctance of doctors to perform a cesarean when deemed in the best interest of the baby and mother.

Also, in the 1960s there was increased emphasis on the welfare of the fetus, and cesarean deliveries were a means of improving fetal outcome.

Many doctors now perform a cesarean as a precautionary measure if there is any risk to the newborn in vaginal delivery. Difficult mid-forceps deliveries are no longer recommended. Many doctors automatically deliver all breech babies by cesarean because of the risks involved in vaginal delivery of a breech baby.

Thus, developments in anesthesia, infection prevention, and surgical techniques have led to a dramatically reduced infant and maternal mortality rate. In many instances a cesarean procedure became the safe means of delivering a healthy baby and preserving the health of the mother. Doctors turned more frequently to the surgical alternative, and the cesarean rate rapidly increased. The rate has now become so high that it is widely criticized.

Statistics demonstrate the sharp increase in the cesarean birth rate. In 1965 5% of all births were by cesareans. By 1975 the rate had leaped to 12% to 15%. In the 80's the cesarean birth rate in the United States has grown to 18% to 20% of all births. Some of the major medical centers reported cesarean rates of 25% or higher.

Two philosophies common in the medical profession help perpetuate the high cesarean rate. One is the general idea that a cesarean section is the ultimate act the obstetrician can perform to ensure the birth of a healthy baby. Second is the old idea "once a cesarean, always a cesarean." Historically, the single most significant factor contributing to the alarming cesarean rate is repeat cesareans, which account for thirty-five percent of all cesareans. The impact of this factor continues to grow. If recent guidelines adopted by the American College of Obstetrics and Gynecology for VBAC's are adopted and implemented by practicing physicians, this trend should be reversed.

In addition to repeat cesareans, other factors have contributed to the recent upsurge in the Cesarean rate. For example, the presence of active genital herpes, which has reached epidemic levels in our country, has become an indication for a first cesarean. This did much to increase the cesarean rate.

Also, women are typically no longer allowed to labor for days. Doctors feel it is safer to perform a cesarean than to subject the mother and baby to the stress of a long and difficult labor. In addition, modern fetal monitoring equipment has led to some increase in the cesarean rate. The fetal monitor detects fetal distress during labor. The course of management for fetal distress may be to intervene surgically.

A major unspoken factor in the continuing high rate of repeat cesarean sections is the management of the physician's time and the avoidance of interruption of his office hours by the unpredictable occurrence of labor, and the convenience of scheduled births to the operating staff at the hospital.

Other reasons sometimes suggested in explanation of the high cesarean rate include: the practice of defensive medicine to avoid malpractice lawsuits, the desire for the higher fees associated with the cesarean delivery, and the lack of residency training in the handling of difficult vaginal births. The validity of such suggestions is problematical, and the extent to which these factors may have contributed to the rising cesarean rate is not known. In a large measure the expanded use of the cesarean section is due to the very low mortality rate associated with this operation. The maternal mortality rate has decreased to almost zero.

The perinatal mortality rate (baby death before, during, or after birth), has fallen to a third of the level experienced three decades ago. Some doctors attribute this to the increased use of the cesarean section. However, recent articles in medical literature discuss institutions which have maintained cesarean rates as low as 5%, even to this day. a rate hard to imagine in the United States. Most of these institutions are foreign hospitals whose perinatal mortality rate has also fallen to a third of the rate of three decades ago. One might conclude, therefore, that factors other than the increased use of cesarean sections are primarily responsible for the lowered rate.

If these perspectives and considerations continue to dictate the standard of care in this country the percentage of cesarean births will continue to escalate. However, if doctors begin to do VBAC's when possible, a significant reduction in the overall cesarean rate will result.

HUMANISM AND MEDICINE

Obviously, great strides have been made in medicine during the last few decades and the experience of Mrs. Bennett, having a cesarean in a Virginia cabin on an operating table made with two planks supported on wine barrels, seems as hard to imagine as an ancient world devoid of technology.

However, although modern medicine made the surgery relatively safe and painless, reduced infant mortality (it is rare today to lose a mother or baby in cesarean birth) and improved the health of the newborn and mother, until very recently nothing had been done by the medical establishment to make the cesarean delivery a warm and human experience—a childbirth experience. Mothers were put to sleep while their babies were born, and fathers were banished from the operating room. None of this did anything to remedy the old misconceptions, anxieties and fears.

As a result, a large number of unhappy cesarean couples have justifiably felt cheated out of a fulfilling childbirth experience. It's easy to understand why prospective parents who talk and daydream for nine months about the birth of their baby, expecting its birth to be a peak experience in their lives, have this dream dashed because the mother must have a cesarean. The father is shooed into a waiting room. He feels afraid for his wife and the unborn baby. He knows nothing about cesareans. He feels powerless, useless, superfluous in the face of this unexpected change of events. He is not in communication with the doctors or his wife during surgery. He feels forgotten, left out, even hurt and angry.

Things are worse yet for his wife, who is trying to adjust to the unnerving news that she is going to have a cesarean, rather than a "normal," delivery. She, too, is uninformed and frightened for herself and the baby. The doctors are busy, her husband has been sent away, and she is alone with her fears and labor pain.

After the surgery is over and the fear has gone, other emotions rush in on the mother. She feels a deep disappointment over the birth experience, as well as a sense of loss and sorrow over losing something cherished that cannot be recovered. This feeling is particularly valid today because families are small and each birth is an event to be particularly anticipated and cherished. She may feel guilty because of her husband's understandable disappointment in not being able to share the natural birth experience. She may also feel a nagging sense of failure. Even if it is a repeat delivery, and the woman knows of the cesarean ahead of time, she may have many of the same negative feelings.

These were the feelings of Nancy Cohen and Gini Fairley, who co-founded C/SEC, Inc. (Cesarean Support, Education, and Concern), in 1973. In 1972, Nancy Cohen underwent an unplanned and unprepared cesarean delivery. Feeling unhappy and confused about her feelings, she wrote to her Lamaze instructor for the names of other couples who had also experienced surprise cesareans. In her letter, Nancy expressed her feelings of disappointment, alienation, and fear in her childbirth experience. She wanted to know if other women felt as she did about their cesarean experience and how there were coping with their emotions.

Her letter was printed in a Lamaze newsletter, which resulted in her receiving mail from cesarean couples from all parts of the country. Gini Fairley was among those who read Nancy's letter. She wrote to Nancy asking that the two of them get together to talk and share their feelings and views on their births.

From their meetings came the mutual resolve to do what they could to make the cesarean delivery a better experience. Other couples joined them, and in 1973 the organization of C/SEC, Inc. was officially formed in Boston. Initially the group was small, but through the collective effort of its members The Boston Hospital for Women was persuaded to change its policy of banning fathers from the operating room. This started a trend that spread to various parts of the country and has been gaining momentum at a rapid pace.

Simultaneously, the work of two other devoted women began in the area of cesarean education. Bonnie Donovan, cesarean mother and author of a contemporary book on cesarean childbirth, *The Cesarean Birth Experience*,[9] and Ruth Allen, nurse, childbirth educator and lecturer, did much to update cesarean education for laypeople and to improve methods of cesarean procedure.

Today, hundreds of cesarean childbirth classes are available to expectant couples. Cesarean education is being added to the regular curriculum of planned childbirth classes such as Lamaze.

Encouraged and inspired by C/SEC, Inc., hundreds of support groups have sprung up all over the country. Some groups are affiliated with C/SEC, Inc., others are not; but all are seeking similar objectives. To illustrate the goals of a support group, we obtained from our local group the following statement of philosophy:

1. We believe that the single most important goal of any childbirth experience is a healthy mother and baby. We feel that our goals are consistent with this belief.

2. We believe the cesarean birth is an alternative method of childbirth, and in most cases, can be, and should be, treated as "the birth of a baby"—a happy, exciting, joyous event—rather than as simply a surgical procedure. We believe that this is possible without losing sight of the fact that it is an operation which must be dealt with seriously and respectfully.

3. We believe cesarean couples have the right to "family-centered" cesarean care. We believe this right can be secured through understanding and communication between cesarean parents, doctors, and their hospitals. The cesarean mother must have available the same newborn care and feeding options as the noncesarean mother. Hospitals and doctors should provide for and support the mother who chooses rooming-in and breastfeeding.

4. We believe [that] through education a cesarean mother will be a happy, confident, relaxed patient, the cesarean couple needs to be fully aware of what to expect from the cesarean delivery, including procedures involved, options that may be available to them, and current research on childbirth. Throughout the hospital stay, the couple has the right to have all questions concerning mother and baby satisfactorily answered.

5. We believe better understanding of the psychological and emotional state of cesarean couples is needed before, during, and after the birth of their child. Parents whose infant has been born by cesarean often have unresolved feelings and questions and have a very real need for this support.

6. We believe that childbirth instructors have a responsibility to include adequate preparation in their classes for cesarean births. Prepared childbirth classes must help to prepare parent [or] parents for whatever childbirth experience may be encountered.

7. We believe that the ideal cesarean birth requires the support of the total medical community and be achieved only with their help.

8. We believe the general public must be made aware of the physical and psychological needs of cesarean couples.[10]

Although the credit for improving the emotional and psychological aspects of the cesarean birth experience (which includes the option for father-attended cesarean birth) largely belongs to a grass-roots movement stemming from the cesarean couples themselves, the improvement is also a result of the efforts of those sincere and dedicated doctors who have supported and promoted an enlightened and shared birth experience for their patients.

Dr. Russell L. Hulme, O.B., and a leading advocate for father-attended cesarean birth sums it up:

> "In our society of human beings, progress must be measured not merely in saving lives and minimizing physical illness, but in enhancing the quality of life, for this affects all of us all the time. The opportunity for improving the quality of life is nowhere greater than in the moments surrounding the most consequential event in our existence—our entrance into this life.
>
> The opportunity for the family unit (mother, father, and newborn infant) to participate together in this monumental event opens the way for establishing a relationship which can transcend all other human experiences and set the course for a vastly improved future for each one. This is where I have witnessed the most significant recent advancements in maternal-child care—in the quality of life of the participants. This is where I have encountered and participated in the most rewarding experiences of my obstetrical career.
>
> The participants in the cesarean birth experience can be assured that the excitement of birth, the thrill at witnessing the newborn infant, the realization of the potential of the baby's existence, the beauty of the family bonding, the opportunity for total involvement, the enhancement of the quality of life for each one be no less fulfilling because of the cesarean experience."[11]

It's been a long and hazardous journey strewn with success and failure, joy and sorrow, from the crude beginnings of cesarean birth to the joyful scene portrayed at the beginning of this chapter. It represents the striving for a better way, a safer, more successful and humanistic way to have a cesarean. At times the changes seem to come painfully slowly. Let's hope that this latest milestone in finding a better way, the pronouncement by the American College of Ostetricians and Gynecologists issuing new guidelines for having a vaginal birth after cesarean, will be implemented immediately. However, history verifies the wisdom of the observation of Niccolo Machiavelli that, "There is nothing more difficult to take in hand, more perilous to conduct, or more uncertain in its success than to take the lead in the introduction of a new order of things."

A recent article appearing in the *American Journal of Obstetrics and Gynecology* states, "Since the risks of a cesarean section include increased maternal mortality and morbidity, we believe informed consent should include the choice of vaginal delivery."

If you are pregnant, qualify for a trial of labor *and* desire one, then request it of your doctor. If he refuses to consider it on the basis that he has never done one, or would prefer to take a wait and see approach to determine what other doctors in the community are doing, or that the hospital at which he primarily practices won't permit a VBAC, then we urge you to seek another doctor. In seeking another physician, check his cesarean section rate and credentials, interview him, and get recommendations before making your choice. We believe that if the mother truly desires a trial of labor her doctor should make arrangements at a hospital (such as a large regional hospital or university center) with an ongoing trial of labor program.

PART II
Before the Birth

CHAPTER THREE

Nutrition

As an expectant mother, you have a strong feeling of responsibility for your unborn baby, and as a result you are probably interested in learning more about nutrition. The unborn baby is totally dependent on your physical well-being. At no other time in its life will your child be in more need of good nourishment as during this nine-month formative period. There is a bond between mother and baby wherein she protects the baby's health by protecting her own.

Studies show that there is a direct relationship between prenatal diet and the lack of complications in pregnancy. A good diet can be instrumental in preventing infection, anemia, and toxemia.

One young mother asked me recently, "Won't the baby just take from my body what it needs? Isn't it true that I am just hurting myself if I don't eat correctly?" It is true that you are hurting yourself by not getting proper nutrition. The fetus will take precious nourishment from your bones and muscles. You aren't being fair to yourself and your family if you allow this to happen, but you are also not being fair to the baby because the baby will get *less* of what he needs this way.* And even this can only happen for a limited time before you both become depleted. Poor nutrition can be very serious for you and disastrous for your unborn baby.

---

*We would have liked to avoid the use of the masculine pronoun for both sexes, but to do so would have been very clumsy in a book of this kind. Therefore, we hope the reader will understand that we intend no sexism, and that we know a baby or a doctor may be *she,* and that a nurse may be *he.* One of the main emphases of this book is that men can share in the birth and care of their own children, even in cesarean births.

Good nutrition benefits the baby in many ways. The foremost benefit is that proper nutrition prevents stillbirths and low birth weight.

Low birth weight (5¹/₂ pounds or less) is more serious than most people realize. It causes about 53,000 infant deaths a year.[1] Low birth weight babies are ten times more likely to suffer from some degree of mental retardation. Studies also indicate that there is a direct relationship between infant birth weight and IQ. The most rapid brain development takes place in the last trimester (three-month period) of pregnancy and also the first month of life. An undernourished mother can be the cause of irreversible neurological damage and permanent brain underdevelopment in her baby.

Breastfeeding also makes many nutritional demands; see Chapter 13 for more information.

WHAT IS A NUTRITIONAL DIET?

A nutritional diet is a diet that supplies each body requirement in the quantity that meets the individual's needs. To plan your diet, you will need to know what the nutrients are, where they come from, and what amounts are needed.

You should select foods that are nutritious and appealing and that keep you in the proper caloric range for one day (2,300–2,400 calories). Remember, you want to gain between twenty-four and thirty pounds by the end of the nine months (see Chapter 4). You should gain this weight at a fairly steady rate. Your doctor or nurse should give you an evaluation of your weight status at the beginning of prenatal care. You should discuss your dietary pattern and your everyday activities to determine a diet and weight gain most suitable for you. You are an individual with a unique background, lifestyle, and preference for food, so you should have a diet tailored to your needs.

FOOD GROUPS[2]

Basically, you need the following each day: four servings of protein, four servings of milk and milk products, four servings of grains, one vitamin C serving (fruit or vegetable), one leafy green vegetable, and one other fruit or vegetable.

Protein Foods

Protein foods include both animal and vegetable foods. Animal foods provide protein, riboflavin, niacin, vitamins B_6 and B_{12}, iron, phosphorus, zinc, and iodine. Vegetable protein foods provide protein, iron, thiamin, folacin (folic acid), vitamins B_6 and E, phosphorus, magnesium, and zinc.

You must have protein four times a day. Protein is the basic material of which most cells are formed. The most complete protein foods are meat, fish, milk, cheese, and eggs. Pregnant women need extra protein to aid the following processes:

1. Rapid growth of the fetus

2. Development of the placenta

3. Enlargement of maternal tissue

4. Increased maternal circulating blood volume

5. Formation of amniotic fluid

6. Storage reserves

Animal Protein Foods.   A serving is 2–3 ounces cooked (boneless) of the following unless otherwise noted.

* Bacon, 6 slices
* Beef: ground, cube, roast, chop
* Canned tuna, salmon, crab, and so on, $1/2$ cup
* Cheese (see section on milk and milk products)
* Clams, 4 large or 9 small
* Eggs, 2
* Fish: filet, steak
* Fish sticks, breaded, 4
* Frankfurters, 2
* Lamb: ground, cube, roast, chop
* Lobster
* Luncheon meat, 3 slices
* Pork, ham: ground, roast, chop
* Poultry: ground, roast
* Sausage links, 4
* Shrimp, scallops, 5–6 large
* Spareribs, 6 medium ribs
* Veal: ground, cube, roast, chop

Vegetable Protein Foods.   A serving is 1 cup cooked unless otherwise stated.

* Canned garbanzo, lima, kidney beans

- Canned pork and beans
- Dried beans and peas
- Lentils
- Peanut butter, $^1/_4$ cup
- Nuts, $^1/_2$ cup
- Sunflower seeds, $^1/_2$ cup
- Tofu (soybean curd)

Milk and Milk Products

Milk and milk products constitute an exchange group for foods containing calcium, phosphorus, vitamin D, and riboflavin. In addition, these foods supply protein, vitamins A, E, B_6, B_{12}, magnesium, and zinc. A serving is 8 ounces (1 cup, or 240 cc) unless otherwise noted. *Note:* Tofu is also a source of calcium; 1 cup of tofu may be exchanged for one serving of the following foods.

- Cheese: hard and semisoft (except blue, Camembert, and cream), $1^1/_2$ oz.
- Cheese spread, 2 oz.
- Cottage cheese, creamed, $1^1/_3$ cups
- Cow's milk: whole, nonfat, low fat, nonfat dry reconstituted, buttermilk
- Cream soups made with milk, 12 oz.
- Evaporated milk, 3 oz.
- Goat's milk (low B_{12} content)
- Ice cream, $1^1/_2$ cups
- Ice milk
- Instant breakfast made with milk, 4 oz.
- Vanilla pudding, custard
- Soybean milk (low B_{12} content)
- Yogurt

Grain Products

Grain products supply thiamin, niacin, riboflavin, iron, phosphorus, and zinc. This exchange group is divided into (1) whole-grain products and (2) enriched products. Enriched breads, cereals, and pastas provide significantly lower amounts of magnesium and zinc than whole-grain products. Whole-grain products are best. *Note:* Pasta, crackers, and bagels can be whole-grain as well as enriched.

Whole-Grain Products.

- Brown rice, $1/2$ cup
- Cereals, hot: oatmeal, rolled wheat, cracked wheat, wheat and malted barley, $1/2$ cup cooked
- Cereals, ready-to-eat: puffed oats, shredded wheat, wheat flakes, granola, $3/4$ cup
- Cracked and whole wheat bread, 1 slice
- Wheat germ, 1 tbsp.

Enriched Breads, Cereals, and Pastas

- Bread, 1 slice
- Cereals, hot: cream of wheat or rice, farina, cornmeal, $1/2$ cup
- Cereals, ready-to-eat, $3/4$ cup
- Corn bread, 2-inch square
- Crackers, 4
- Pasta, $1/2$ cup
- Muffin, biscuit, dumpling 1
- Pancake, 1 medium
- Rice, cooked, $1/2$ cup
- Roll or bagel, 1
- Tortillas, corn, 2
- Tortilla, flour, 1 large
- Waffle, 1 large

Vitamin C Sources

Vitamin C-rich fruits and vegetables supply ascorbic acid. Fresh, frozen, or canned forms may be used, although the vitamin C content of canned products is lower.

Juices

- Orange, grapefruit, 4 oz.
- Tomato, pineapple, 12 oz.
- Fruit juices and drinks enriched with vitamin C, 6 oz.

Fruits

- Cantaloupe, $1/2$
- Grapefruit, $1/2$
- Guava, $1/4$ medium

- Mango, 1 medium
- Orange, 1 medium
- Papaya, $1^1/_3$ medium
- Strawberries, $^3/_4$ cup
- Tangerines, 2 small

Vegetables

- Bok choy, $^3/_4$ cup
- Broccoli, 1 stalk
- Brussels sprouts, 3–4
- Cabbage, cooked, $1^1/_3$ cups
- Cauliflower, raw or cooked, 1 cup
- Greens (collards, kale, mustard, turnip): $^3/_4$ cup
- Peppers, chili, $^3/_4$ cup
- Peppers: green, red, $^1/_2$ medium
- Tomatoes, 2 medium
- Watercress, $^3/_4$ cup

Leafy Vegetables

Leafy green vegetables form an exchange group for folacin (folic acid). In addition, these foods supply vitamins A, E, and B_6, riboflavin, iron, and magnesium. A serving is 1 cupful raw, or $^3/_4$ cup cooked.

- Asparagus
- Bok choy
- Broccoli
- Brussels sprouts
- Cabbage
- Dark leafy lettuce (for example, romaine, not iceberg)
- Scallions
- Watercress

Other Fruits and Vegetables

Other fruits and vegetables include yellow fruits and vegetables that supply significant amounts of vitamin A. Vitamin A is also found in outstanding amounts in the leafy green vegetable group. Other fruits and vegetables also contribute varying amounts of B-complex vitamins, vitamin E, magnesium, zinc, and phosphorus. A serving is $^1/_2$ cup (fresh, frozen, or canned) unless otherwise indicated.

Vegetables

- Artichokes
- Bamboo shoots
- Bean sprouts: alfalfa, mung
- Beets
- Carrots
- Cauliflower
- Celery
- Corn
- Cucumber
- Eggplant
- Beans: green, wax
- Hominy
- Lettuce
- Mushrooms
- Nori seaweed
- Onions
- Parsnips
- Peas
- Pea pods
- Potatoes
- Radishes
- Summer squash, winter squash, zucchini
- Sweet potatoes

Fruits

- Apricot, fresh, 1 large
- Nectarines, 2 medium
- Peach, fresh, 1 medium
- Persimmon, 1 small
- Prunes, 4 (also a significant iron source)
- Pumpkin, 1/4 cup
- Apple, 1 medium
- Banana, 1 small
- Cherries
- Berries
- Dates, 5

- Figs, 2 large
- Fruit cocktail
- Grapes
- Kumquats, 3
- Pear, 1 medium
- Pineapple
- Plums, 2 medium
- Raisins (also significant iron source)
- Watermelon

A DAY'S SAMPLE MENU

Some women find it helpful to have a sample menu to follow. For this reason, we have provided the following menu.[3]

Breakfast	Orange juice Bran flakes with peaches Milk
Morning Snack	Peanut butter and jelly on whole wheat toast Glass of milk Pear
Lunch	Glass of vegetable juice Egg salad on lettuce Two slices of pumpernickel bread Tomato slices
Afternoon Snack	Cup of yogurt Carrot sticks Glass of water or other beverage
Dinner	Chicken Carrot-raisin-apple salad Whole baked potato Green peas Glass of apple juice
Evening Snack	Crackers with cheese Glass of milk Dried apricots

KEY NUTRIENTS

The following chart summarizes the key nutrients and the reasons why each is needed and identifies foods that are good sources of each nutrient. It is a guide to understanding why you need to eat a wide variety of foods to be well nourished and healthy.

Key Nutrients

Nutrient	Why Needed	Some Important Sources
Protein	• Builds and maintains all tissues • Forms an important part of enzymes, hormones, and body fluids • Supplies energy	Top-quality protein for tissue building and repair found in lean meat, poultry, fish, seafoods, eggs, milk, and cheese; dry beans, peas, and nuts next best; Cereals, bread, fruits and vegetables also provide some protein but of lower quality
Carbohydrates	• Supply energy from food • Help body use fat efficiently • Spare protein to help in body building and repair	Starches: breads, cereals, corn, grits, potatoes, rice, spaghetti, macaroni and noodles. Sugar: honey, molasses, syrups
Fats	• Supply food energy in compact form (weight for weight supplies twice as much energy as carbohydrates) • Some supply essential fatty acids • Help body use certain other nutrients	Cooking fats and oils, butter, margarine, salad dressings, and oils
Calcium	• Builds bones and teeth • Helps blood to clot • Helps nerves, muscles, and heart to function properly	Milk—whole, skim, buttermilk; fresh, dried, canned; cheese—and leafy vegetables, such as collards, dandelion, kale, mustard and turnip greens
Thiamine	• Helps body cells obtain energy from food • Helps keeps nerves in healthy condition • Promotes good appetite and digestion	Lean pork, heart, kidney, liver, dry beans and peas; whole grain and enriched cereals and breads, and some nuts
Riboflavin	• Helps cells use oxygen to release energy from food • Helps keep eyes healthy • Helps keep skin around mouth and nose smooth	Milk, liver, kidney, heart, lean meat, eggs, and dark leafy greens
Iodine	• Helps the thyroid gland to work properly	Iodized salt; saltwater fish and other seafood
Niacin	• Helps body cells use oxygen to produce energy • Helps maintain health of skin, tongue, digestive tract, and nervous system	Liver, yeast, lean meat, poultry, fish, leafy greens, peanuts and peanut butter, beans and peas, and whole grain and enriched breads and cereals

Key Nutrients (continued)

Nutrient	Why Needed	Some Important Sources
Iron	• Combines with protein to make hemoglobin, the red substance of blood that carries oxygen from the lungs to muscles, brain, and other parts of the body • Helps cells use oxygen	Liver, kidney, heart, oysters, lean meat, egg yolk, dry beans, dark-green leafy vegetables; dried fruit; whole grain and enriched breads and cereals, and molasses
Vitamin A	• Helps eyes adjust to dim light • Helps keep skin smooth • Helps keep lining of mouth, nose, throat, and digestive tract healthy and resistent to infection • Promotes growth	Liver; dark-green and deep-yellow vegetables such as broccoli, turnip and other leafy greens, carrots, pumpkin, sweet potatoes, winter squash; apricots, cantaloupe; butter, fortified margarine
Vitamin C (ascorbic acid)	• Helps hold body cells together and strengthens walls of blood vessels • Helps heal wounds • Helps form teeth and bone	Cantaloupe, grapefruit, oranges, strawberries, broccoli, brussels sprouts, raw cabbage, collards, green and sweet red peppers, mustard and turnip greens, potatoes cooked in jacket, and tomatoes
Vitamin D	• Helps body use calcium and phosphorus to build strong bones and teeth—important in growing children and during pregnancy and lactation	Fish liver oils; foods fortified with vitamin D, such as milk; direct sunlight produces vitamin D from cholesterol in the skin
Water	• Important part of all body cells and fluids • Carries nutrients to and waste from body cells • Aids in digestion and absorption of food • Helps regulate body temperature	Water, beverages, soup, fruits, and vegetables; most foods contain some water

Source: Adapted from *Key Nutrients*, PA–691, Federal Extension Service, USDA, Washington, D.C.

VEGETARIAN DIETS

There are many advantages to a vegetarian diet. If you are a vegetarian, you are probably not overweight; you avoid overprocessed, empty-calorie food; and your foods have high water and fiber content, low fat content, virtually no cholesterol, and a high polyunsaturated-saturated fat ratio.

Despite these advantages, you must be aware of certain potential nutrient problems. The complete vegetarian diet (omitting all milk and milk products) does not contain any significant amount of vitamin B_{12}. Lacto-ovo vegetarians (who drink milk and eat eggs) can obtain the recommended dietary allowance for this vitamin by drinking the equivalent of four glasses of cow's milk daily. But if you drink only *soybean* and / or *goat's* milk, you will need to take a vitamin B_{12} supplement. A deficiency of vitamin B_{12} causes anemia and eventually results in spinal cord degeneration. A high intake of folacin (such as in prescribed prenatal vitamin pills) will hide this anemia, and thus vitamin B_{12} deficiency may go undiagnosed. The irreversible neurological changes will then be the first indication of a deficiency.[4]

Protein is not a problem in a vegetarian diet if you eat plenty of calories and a *wide variety* of plant proteins. If your diet is below 2,300 to 2,400 calories, your body will use the protein for energy instead of for growth and maintenance. It's a good idea to keep high-

Complementary Plant Protein Sources

Food	Amino Acids Deficient	Complementary Protein
Grains	Isoleucine Lysine	Rice + legumes Corn + legumes Wheat + legumes Wheat + peanut + milk Wheat + sesame + soybean Rice + sesame Rice + brewer's yeast
Legumes	Tryptophan Methionine	Legumes + rice Beans + wheat Beans + corn Soybeans + rice + wheat Soybeans + corn + milk Soybeans + wheat + sesame Soybeans + peanuts + sesame Soybeans + peanuts + wheat + rice Soybeans + sesame + wheat
Nuts and Seeds	Isoleucine Lysine	Peanuts + sesame + soybeans Sesame + beans Sesame + soybeans + wheat Peanuts + sunflower seeds
Vegetables	Isoleucine Methionine	Lima beans Green peas Brussels sprouts } + sesame seeds or Brazil nuts or mushrooms Cauliflower Broccoli Greens + millet or converted rice

protein snacks around, such as peanut butter with crackers, soybeans, or cottage cheese with corn chips.

Amino acids are used by the body to make protein. Unlike animal foods, most plant foods do not have all the essential amino acids in the appropriate amounts, are referred to as "incomplete," and cannot be used to build body tissue. However, by combining several plant foods you can obtain a usable combination. Eaten at the same meal, a correct combination of incomplete proteins makes a complete protein that your body can then use.

Perhaps you are not eating much meat, not because you are a vegetarian, but because the high cost of meat exceeds your food budget. There are low-cost, high-protein foods you can buy to supplement meat. For instance, noninstant powdered skim milk is a good and inexpensive source of protein. Also, peanut butter, cottage cheese, American or Swiss cheese, wheat germ, and soybeans are excellent substitutes. If you are pregnant, you may be wise to budget more of your income for nutritious food. In addition to assuring a healthier baby, nutritious food is low in cost compared to the medical costs resulting from improper nutrition.

THE NEED FOR PRENATAL VITAMINS

Most prenatal care includes a multivitamin pill to be taken daily. Many authorities state that you do not need to take prenatal vitamins if you are eating a nutritious diet every day, without exception. However, there are two important nutrient needs that cannot be met through diet and that are essential to your health and that of the baby. You need a daily supplement of iron and of folacin (folic acid). The growing fetus is building its own blood supply. Your body is making new red blood cells as its fluid and blood volume increases. Without these vital nutrients, you may get anemia.

The daily multivitamin pill may give you a false sense of security that all your nutritional needs are being met. Not all the essential nutrients are contained in these supplements. Your best source of vitamins and minerals is nutritious, carefully prepared (not overcooked) food.

Do not make the mistake of thinking "If multivitamins are good for me, more will be better." An excess of vitamins may be related to birth defects and can be damaging to your kidneys and liver.

You should not take any medication, not even an aspirin, without consulting your doctor.

There are many foods you should avoid. Be careful of artificial substances such as BHA and BHT. These preservatives are found in almost all snack chips, sausage meat, various cake mixes, and even in most cold cereals and some canned foods. These chemicals accumulate in body fat, and the safety of their long-term use hasn't been proven. Therefore, eat sparingly, if at all, of foods that have been processed with BHA or BHT.[5] In general, avoid excessive use of salt, sugar, white flour, soft drinks, coffee, and tea. The caffeine in coffee and tea is not healthful. The question of whether caffeine causes birth defects in humans is far from settled, but the results of many studies prove that large doses of caffeine may harm the baby.

When you go to the market, get in the habit of reading labels. This will tell you what ingredients are in the product. It will help you discover hidden sugar and determine which brand is most nutritious. The ingredients are listed by quantity: the main ingredient listed first, the least ingredient listed last. Finally, remember that food should be properly stored and not overcooked.

DIURETICS AND THE IMPORTANCE OF SALT IN YOUR DIET

In the past, salt and sodium were often routinely restricted in a pregnant woman's diet. New research now indicates that this restriction can be hazardous. During pregnancy, the requirement for sodium is believed to be increased. It is needed to maintain normal levels of sodium in your plasma, muscle, bone, and brain during the large increase in your blood volume and tissue (your body fluid almost doubles). Many women are in the habit of taking diuretics to keep the swelling down or to reduce body fluid. This habit is extremely dangerous to you unless prescribed by your physician. There may be situations where it can be beneficial; let your physician be your guide in this important area.

To ensure getting enough sodium, lightly salt your food and let your taste buds be your guide. Use iodized, not sea, salt. Iodine is an essential mineral that is not present in sea salt.

AVOID SMOKING DURING PREGNANCY

Many things beside foods may adversely affect the unborn baby. Cigarette smoking is one of the biggest offenders. Studies have proven that the level of lead in the blood vessels of an unborn baby increases in proportion to the level found in the baby's smoking mother. Also, toxic substances from cigarette smoke such as carbon monoxide and cyanide retard fetal growth. Smokers tend to have smaller babies than women who do not smoke.

If you smoke, you increase the requirement for most nutrients and at the same time decrease your natural appetite. The amount of vitamin C in your blood drops drastically, leaving you and the baby vulnerable to infections and possible abnormalities.

If you have ever considered quitting smoking, surely now is the time to stop. This is easier said than done. If you need professional help, write to any of the following agencies. Consult your local telephone directory for listings of local chapters (starred items).

*American Cancer Society
777 3rd Avenue
New York, NY 10017

*American Heart Association
1720 Greenville Avenue
Dallas, TX 75231

General Headquarters
5-Day Plan to Stop Smoking
*Seventh Day Adventist Church
Narcotics Education Division
6840 Eastern Avenue, N.W.
Washington, DC 20012

*American Lung Association
1740 Broadway
New York, NY 10019

National Interagency Council on Smoking and Health
Room 1005
291 Broadway
New York, NY 10007

Schick Laboratories
1901 Avenue of the Stars, Suite 1530
Los Angeles, CA 90067

*SmokeEnders
Memorial Parkway
Phillipsburg, NJ 18864

Office on Smoking and Health
U.S. Department of Health, Education, and Welfare
Room 1–58
5600 Fishers Lane
Rockville, MD 20857

Office of Cancer Communications
National Cancer Institute
National Institutes of Health
Bethesda, MD 20205

ALCOHOL USE IN PREGNANCY

Alcohol is also harmful to the unborn baby. Our society takes alcohol for granted, so most people forget that it is a drug. Yet wine, gin and tonic, beer—all alcoholic drinks—contain a central nervous system depressant that affects nearly all our organs. Heavy drinking of alcohol can lead to many serious problems, including muscle and heart diseases, digestive problems, malnutrition, and cirrhosis of the liver. And drinking alcohol during pregnancy can also harm your delicate unborn baby.

What Heavy Drinking Does to the Unborn Baby

The results of recent studies on infants born to women who drank heavily during pregnancy are disturbing. Many babies showed a definite pattern of physical, mental, and behavioral abnormalities that researchers named the "fetal alcohol syndrome." Such babies were abnormally short and light in weight, and even special postnatal care did not help them catch up. Their heads were abnormally small; their faces, joints, limbs, and hearts were malformed, and they were poorly coordinated. Many were hyperactive, extremely nervous, and inattentive. Some were born without these characteristics, while others showed only some features of the syndrome.

How can alcohol so devastate the unborn baby? When a pregnant woman drinks alcohol, it passes through the placenta to the fetus in the same concentration as in the mother's bloodstream. If the mother-to-be gets drunk, her baby gets drunk too. But the baby can't handle alcohol nearly as well as its mother can. For example, the baby's undeveloped liver burns up alcohol less than half as fast as an adult liver can, so the alcohol stays in the baby longer. Unfortunately, an unborn baby can't say no when it's had enough.

Alternatives to Alcohol

All pregnant women feel some stress. And some women feel more anxiety and depression than usual during pregnancy. Sometimes a little alcohol may seem like a good way to shake off that stress. But there are other ways you can handle such feelings.

First, what exactly is bothering you? Could you take some specific action to improve the situation? Would talking to a friend help? Exercise, listening to music, or doing something creative like gardening or painting, help relieve stress. Meditation, pounding a pillow to vent frustration, and writing out your feelings can also be very effective alternatives to alcohol.

Other drugs are *not* an alternative to alcohol. People who are seriously depressed or anxious and can't seem to shake it off should consider asking for outside help. Women's centers often run counseling programs and special support groups. You can get the names of counselors from women's centers, mental health agencies, and your own doctor. If you are drinking too much, get help from a local council on alcoholism, mental health agency, Alcoholics Anonymous, or Women for Sobriety group. Most such groups are listed in local telephone directories.

There are many restrictions associated with pregnancy, and sometimes they may seem overwhelming. There is so much advice and so many recommendations. But it is important that you understand that your actions *do* make a difference to your unborn baby. If you avoid alcohol during pregnancy, you *do* give your baby a better chance in life.

For further information, write

National Clearinghouse for Alcohol Information
Box 2345
Rockville, MD 20852

National Institute on Alcohol Abuse and Alcoholism
5600 Fishers Lane
Rockville, MD 20857

U.S. Department of Health, Education, and Welfare
Public Health Service
Alcohol, Drug Abuse, and Mental Health Administration
Washington, DC 20201

OTHER DRUGS

Marijuana and such drugs as LSD, heroin, cocaine, amphetamines, and barbiturates should be strictly avoided in pregnancy. Women who have drug habits should get professional help. Don't be afraid to tell your doctor you use marijuana or other drugs just because you think the doctor will disapprove of what you are doing. If you don't want to tell your own doctor, make an appointment with another doctor to discuss this problem. You also might call a "hot line" or a drug clinic for help.

Dr. Cherilyn Sheets warns, "Certain medication, including some antibiotics, such as tetracycline, and tranquilizers can be dangerous. If a pregnant woman takes tetracycline during the last half of her pregnancy, it may result in gray stains on the baby's teeth when they grow in.[6] When this adverse reaction to tetracycline came to the attention of the FDA (Federal Drug Administration) the agency warned physicians not to prescribe tetracycline in any form for expectant mothers or children under eight years of age, unless other drugs were not likely to be effective. However, the July 1978 to June 1979 National Disease and Therapeutic Index shows that 60 percent of the prescriptions for liquid tetracycline are written for children under ten years old.[7]

The stains from tetracycline are permanent. If your doctor gives you an antibiotic, examine the lable. If it is tetracycline, ask your doctor if another drug would be just as effective.

NUTRITION AND SURGERY

Because you will be experiencing a surgical birth, it is even more important to be in the best nutritional state, because this will make surgery and the recovery process easier for you. Surgery is an enormous stress to your body, and you want to be in the best possible shape to cope with its effects. Your nutritional state will affect things such as the ability of your blood to clot, how readily your blood can carry vital nutrients (such as oxygen) to the site of surgical incision, your body's ability to cope with both physical and emotional stress, and how rapidly your body heals itself. Remember, the doctor sews up the incision, but your body mends it by making new cells. That repairing process is directly related to the food you put into your body. That old saying, "You are what you eat," is profound and true.

CHAPTER FOUR

Weight Gain in Pregnancy

A question that invariably comes up in our cesarean childbirth classes from a mother with older children is "Why did my doctor tell me I had to keep my weight under twenty pounds with my previous pregnancies, and now he tells me I should gain a minimum of twenty-four pounds?" In the recent past, it was believed that the baby's birth weight was not related to the mother's weight gain during pregnancy. Also, a gain of more than twenty pounds put an undue and sudden strain on the mother's legs and back. Certain serious complications such as preeclampsia and eclampsia convulsions caused by a toxic condition were less common in women with a moderate weight gain.*

And, last, weight gain in pregnancy seemed to be additive with each successive pregnancy. If a mother was interested in retaining her figure and health, she was advised to limit her weight gain to as little as fifteen pounds. Doctors stressed limiting weight gain, and women were fearful when they stepped on that scale each month at the doc-

---

*Preeclampsia and eclampsia are toxic conditions that, although rare, may occur during the last three months of pregnancy. Preeclampsia is the forerunner of eclampsia and is characterised by a sudden rise in blood pressure, albumen (protein) in the urine, and swelling of the face and fingers. When the condition becomes so severe that convulsions and coma occur, it is called *eclampsia*. The exact cause is unknown, although it is related to being pregnant.

tor's office. Women would starve themselves for a few days prior to their checkup each month.

The profound turnabout in thinking about the ideal weight gain in pregnancy results from recent studies in the field of prenatal nutrition, showing that the mother's weight gain has a profound influence on pregnancy outcome. Studies have now shown that women who gain an average of thirty pounds during pregnancy usually have babies averaging seven to eight pounds at birth. Seven- to eight-pound babies are easier to care for than five-pound babies. They are more vigorous, active, and mentally alert and suffer less from colic, diarrhea, anemia, and infections.

There is also new evidence that children of low weight at birth have more health problems, more hospitalization for illness and more learning problems when they later enter school than babies of average weight. Pregnant women are now being advised to gain a minimum of twenty-four pounds, and underweight women may be advised to gain up to forty pounds.[1] Overweight women must be doubly cautious to eliminate any junk food from their diet and make sure that everything they eat is nutritious. They will not be advised to diet. *This is not the time for anyone to diet. Starve yourself and you are literally starving the baby.* Weight-reducing programs should not be used during pregnancy. If you restrict your weight you increase the risk of having an unhealthy baby. Dieting can, in extreme cases, result in infant mortality. When a pregnant woman reduces her intake of calories, her body will use the protein that the baby needs for growth and for its own energy supply.

An example of the danger of dieting while pregnant can be seen in the documented case of a thirty-one-year-old woman who was director of research for the House Banking and Currency Committee in Washington, D.C. She entered her second pregnancy in 1979 with a normal obstetric history and in good health. She had started her first pregnancy at 120 pounds. She had attended Lamaze classes in the Washington, D.C., area and delivered a 6-pound 15-ounce boy.

Seven months later, she conceived again, at which time her weight was 135 pounds. It is not known whether her obstetrician counseled her as to weight gain or nutrition during pregnancy. Her husband became concerned because she ate so little early in the second pregnancy. Between her fifth and sixth months of pregnancy, she gained only 1 pound. However, in her seventh month she suddenly gained 9 pounds due to marked edema (swelling caused by water retention). She had to have her rings cut off. Later she developed severe abdominal pains. While she was being x-rayed for possible appendicitis, she went into convulsions. She was taken to surgery and delivered a stillborn baby weighing 2 pounds 9 ounces. The woman died after several days of intensive care. It was discovered after her death that she had been following a popular rapid weight loss diet.[2]

This incident was an extreme case. However, a survey of women entering prenatal classes in four geographic areas of the United States reported that between 24 and 79 percent of women entering such classes were actually dieting to hold the line at their seventh-month weight gains. Moreover, up to 66 percent of these women were told nothing by their doctors regarding an ideal weight gain. Of those who had been given a recommended weight gain, as many as 10 percent thought the gain prescribed was too high. In addition, 7 percent of the women surveyed were actually trying to lose weight.[3]

Women should be aware that the third trimester (last three months) is the time of maximal fetal brain tissue development, and the baby also develops a protective layer of fat, adding several pounds. Not only does the fetus rely on continued maternal weight gain, but the mother's own blood volume must also be protected by the daily consumption of 2,200 to 2,600 calories and at least 75 grams of protein. (One quart of milk and two eggs supply about 40 grams of protein.)[4]

Thus, even if you gain twenty-four pounds during the first six months of your pregnancy, you should still continue to gain up to a little less than one pound per week. Do not diet just because you think you have gained your total allowed weight, because most of the baby's weight will be gained during the last three months. *Do* eliminate all empty calories—cookies, cakes, pudding, and so on.

Doctors and mothers alike are beginning to appreciate more and more that the components and rate of weight gain are more important than the actual number of pounds a woman gains. The *quality* of the weight gain is crucial. Gaining too much fat or fluid won't help you or the baby. The desirable thing is to gain from nutritional food at a steady rate. Don't worry if in your current pregnancy you are gaining at a somewhat different rate from the rate at which you gained in a previous one, or at a different rate from that of a friend. Every woman is different, and every pregnancy is different. Your doctor will be charting your weight gain and will be able to advise you.

The range of weight gain recommended by your doctor will be related to the following characteristics associated with your pregnant state:

Characteristic	Weight
Fetus	$7^1/_2$ to $8^1/_2$ lb (average newborn weight)
Placenta	1 or 2 lbs
Amniotic fluid	1 or 2 lbs
Increases in Mother's Blood and Body Fluid	4 to 8 lbs
Uterine muscles	2 to 3 lbs
Breast increase	2 to 3 lbs
Fat deposits	2 to 10 lbs

Source: Adapted from T. Hotchner, *Pregnancy and Childbirth* (New York: Avon, 1979), p. 67.

The average immediate weight loss at birth is usually 13 pounds —this includes the baby, amniotic fluid, and the placenta. Usually another $3^1/_2$ pounds are lost in the next two days, mostly water lost from your body tissue. More weight is lost during the next six weeks as your body returns to its prepregnant state. If you still find yourself overweight, the rest will gradually be lost depending on your food intake, activity, and body metabolism.

FETAL DEVELOPMENT

Where does all that nutrition go? What is taking shape inside you? Most mothers are intensely curious about the fetus as it develops. Each month as the mother's body shape is changing, she wonders about the baby. How much does it weigh? What does it look like? The following is a general description of what is taking place. You may enjoy referring to this chart each month as your pregnancy progresses.

Development of the Embryo

End of First Month

The embryo, having passed the microscopic stage, is now a small, visible dot of tissue.

Second Month

The embryo is now about one inch long. The head and limbs are partially formed. It is recognizable as an infant.

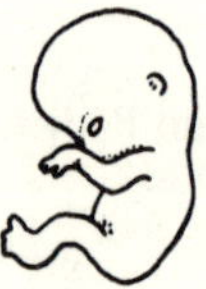

Third Month

The limbs, little fingers, toes, and ears are fully formed. Fingernails and toenails are beginning to appear. The sex can be distinguished. The fetus now weighs about 1 ounce and is approximately 3 inches long.

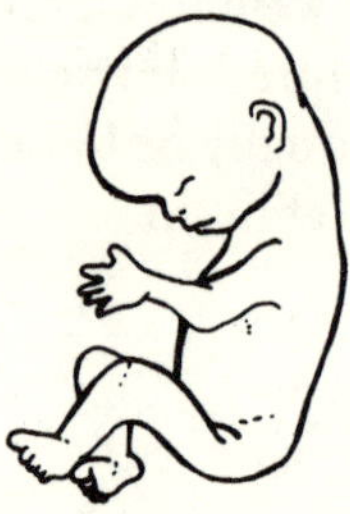

Fourth Month

The fetus now weighs about $1/2$ pound and is approximately 8 inches long. The skin is a pinkish color and is covered with soft, fine hair. Hair forming eyebrows and eyelashes is visible. The doctor can usually detect a heartbeat by now. The bone structure of the infant can be detected by x-ray. The most exciting thing is that you may now begin to feel the baby move!

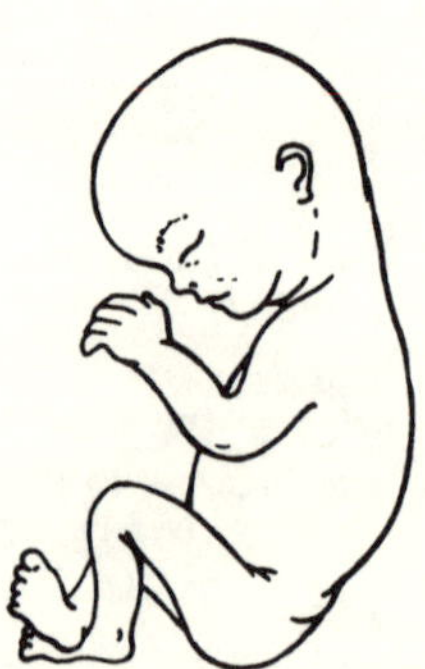

Fifth Month

About 12 inches long and weighing about 1 pound, the baby now has hair on its head.

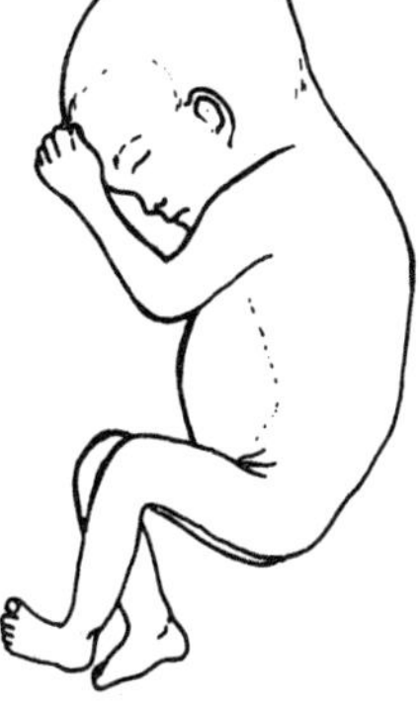

Sixth Month

Now 14 inches long and weighing about 2 pounds, the baby resembles a wrinkled old man.

Seventh Month

Approximately 16 inches long and weighing about 3 pounds, the baby now has accumulated a little more fat under the skin and is more attractive.

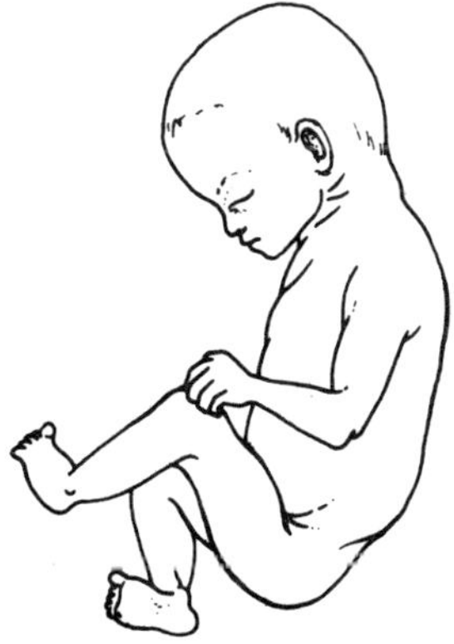

Eighth Month

The baby is now about 18 inches long and weighs about 5 pounds. The chances of survival if born now are generally good.

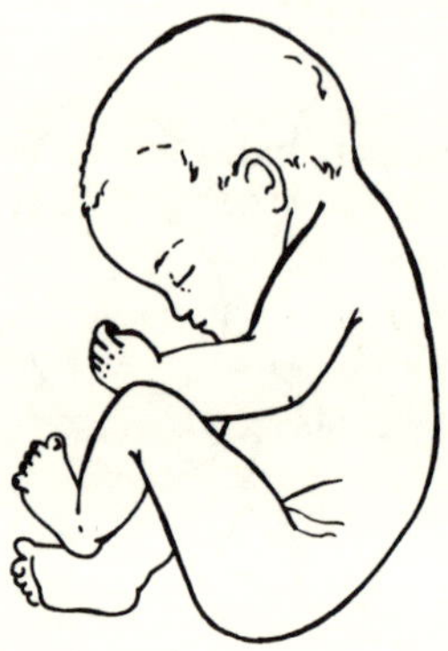

Ninth Month

On the average, the baby now will be about 20 inches in length and weigh about 8 pounds. The baby's skin is almost smooth now and is covered with a cheeselike material. The head is as large as the shoulders are wide.

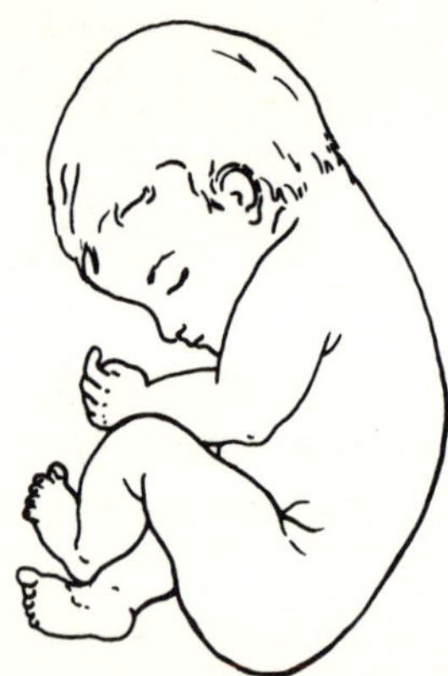

Now that you understand where and why the twenty-five to thirty-five pounds are needed for a healthy pregnancy, relax and don't starve yourself. Eat sensibly. Follow your doctor's advice concerning your diet and weight gain.

CHAPTER FIVE

Exercise and Mobility

Regular exercise will be beneficial to you during your pregnancy. Exercise helps reduce tension and promotes increased circulation, resulting in a feeling of well-being. However, if you were not in the habit of exercising before you became pregnant, do not begin any exercise program without first consulting with your doctor.

Walking might be the ideal exercise for you. Walking helps digestion, circulation, and relaxation and promotes good muscle tone. When walking, it's a good idea to take it easy at first and gradually build up distance. An evening walk with your husband and children can be very relaxing and pleasant for everyone.

If you are the athletic type and are involved in exercise programs and sports, you should be able to continue these activities for as long as they are comfortable. Swimming, for example, is an excellent sport for pregnant women. It uses many muscles with little chance of strain or accident. Jogging, however, is not recommended because it is hard on your breasts and back. During pregnancy, the hormone progesterone relaxes the ligaments in your back. If the ligaments are stretched, they may not go back to their prior shape after pregnancy.

Exercises that pull on the abdominal muscles, such as sit-ups, are also not a good idea. The longitudinal muscles of your abdomen separate in the middle to allow room for your expanding uterus. Sit-ups encourage this separation even more. Experts suggest that this may delay the recovery of abdominal tone after delivery.

It's a good idea to exercise for short periods of time and never to the point of fatigue. When you are pregnant, your energy reserve is reduced. It may take a nonpregnant woman half an hour to recover from fatigue, but it may take you half a day.

SUGGESTED PRENATAL EXERCISES

If you want to condition your body try the following exercises. Start your exercise program gradually. Do a few exercises each day, and as you begin to strengthen your muscles, you will soon be surprised at how much lighter your baby feels.

Be sure to take a deep "cleansing" breath before each exercise. Also remember to breathe deeply as you exercise. Breathe in as you relax, and exhale during the difficult part of the exercise. While you are exercising, your body needs extra oxygen for your muscles and to help you relax.

1. *To strengthen abdominal and back muscles*

   a. Lie on your back on a hard surface. Point your toes. Raise your right leg slightly and stretch your left arm toward the raised leg. Relax the arm and leg, and repeat with the opposite arm and leg. Repeat exercise five times.

   b. Lie on your back with your knees bent and your feet flat on the floor. Tilt your pelvis by pressing your lower back flat against the ground. At the same time, tighten your abdominal muscles and tuck in your buttocks. Keep your knees and thighs together. Relax your back. Repeat exercise five times.

   c. Lie on your back and slowly raise your right leg as high as you can, keeping your left leg straight on the floor. Bend your foot toward you and slowly lower your leg, keeping your knees straight. Repeat with left leg. Raise each leg three times.

2. *To strengthen inner and outer thigh muscles and back muscles.* Lie on your side. With one hand, support your head, with the other hand support your body on the ground. Flex your feet, tighten your buttocks and abdominal muscles. Raise your upper leg slowly as high as you can. Now slowly lower the leg, bringing it in line with the resting leg. Remember to keep your abdominal and buttock muscles tightened. Repeat with the other leg.

3. *To strengthen abdominal muscles and improve circulation and leg flexibility.* Lie on your back with your arms outstretched. Bend both legs at the knees and bring your legs off the floor, keeping your back flat on the floor. Press your knees tightly together, and move your legs rapidly up and down ten times.

4. *To improve posture and strengthen back.* Stand with your feet flat on the floor. Stand tall, with your body in good alignment. Now relax your back and bend forward slowly, curving your back

and relaxing arms and neck. Then raise your back up *slowly,* so that you feel each vertebra, until you are standing tall again.

5. *To keep back flexible and ease backache.* Sit with your knees bent and feet flat on the ground. Curve your back, relax your arms over your knees, and drop your head forward. Then slowly straighten your back. Repeat five times.

6. *Back and trunk exercise.* Stand with your arms stretched straight out, feet flat on the ground. Bend to your left and move your right arm over your head. Stretch forward with both arms (keep your back straight). Now stretch to the right with your left arm raised over your head. Repeat in opposite direction. Straighten up and take a deep breath.

MOBILITY: MOVING THROUGH THE DAY

Alas, there comes a time in the last months of pregnancy when your stomach is so big that doing exercises or participating in sports leaves you wondering whether to laugh or cry. One pregnant woman relates that she was determined to play tennis every day, as was her custom, until she was scheduled to go to the hospital. She was eight months pregnant, and in her tennis clothes she looked like a volleyball with arms and legs. Nevertheless, her enthusiasm was not diminished. She would get out there and play her best. One afternoon, during a tough match, she was running for a ball when she felt a gush of fluid drench her tennis shorts and run down her legs. "My bag of water has broken," she wailed, "Get me to the hospital." Quickly her tennis partner rushed her to her doctor's office. The doctor gave her a quick exam. He couldn't help laughing as he said, "I'll bet you haven't had an accident like this since you were potty trained." The pressure of the baby on her bladder had caused her to urinate without even realizing it. That was the last game of tennis for this lady until after the baby was born.

Tennis and sports aside, the pregnant woman will find when her tummy becomes large most movements are awkward, difficult, or downright impossible. With a big abdomen in the way, little things such as turning over in bed, getting out of a chair, bending, lifting, and carrying things sometimes require imagination and effort. You must be careful not to hurt yourself. It is very easy to hurt your back if you lift heavy objects incorrectly. The following helpful hints, are adapted from Elizabeth Bing's popular book entitled, *Moving Through Pregnancy*.[1] She offered to let us share them with you.

Getting out of Bed

The first maneuver to figure out each day is how to get you and your ten-pound tummy out of bed successfully. Try this: Bend your legs and roll over onto your side. Push yourself up into a sitting position with your hands. Now rotate your feet to get the blood circulating. To avoid getting leg cramps, don't stretch your feet or point your toes, while you are still lying down. Instead, when you are sitting up, pull your toes toward you and gently stretch your legs. Swing your legs over the side of the bed and stand up.

Check Your Posture

Working on good posture is one of the best things you can do for your body. As you stand up, develop the habit of checking your posture. Stretch the top of your head, and check your body alignment. To check your posture, stand with hips firmly pressed against a wall and your feet together, knees slightly flexed and heels six to eight inches from the wall. Press your shoulders and back against the wall, trying to eliminate the space at the small of your back. Pull in your lower abdominal muscles and tuck in your buttocks. Check how this posture feels, and try to maintain it during the day. You can also do this check against the floor while lying on your back with your knees bent.

Putting on Stockings

Even putting on stockings can be a task when your tummy sticks out as far as your elbows! Try putting your right foot on a chair that is slightly to the right of you. As you bend toward the foot to put your stocking on, your big abdomen is as little in your way as possible. You will feel well supported on your standing left leg as well as on your right leg, which is resting on the chair. Straighten up as you pull your stockings up.

Putting on Your Shoes

Putting shoes on can be equally trying. Sit with your legs well apart. Bend over your abdomen and pull on your shoes. Or, pull your right leg up, rest it on your left knee, and put on the shoe.

Squat to Lift Objects

Lift heavy objects by squatting, not by bending over. Squatting may not look very ladylike, but it works. To squat, put your weight on your toes, and keep your knees well apart to make room for your abdomen. To get up, straighten your legs, lock your knees (with your trunk still bending forward), then straighten up your trunk. Rising while straightening your legs and back at the same time puts too much of a strain on your thigh muscles.

Working in the Kitchen

When standing at the kitchen sink, your growing abdomen always seems to get in the way. There is a tendency to overcompensate with a hollow back. Check your posture: Straighten your back and tuck your tail in. This will allow you to get closer to the sink and will put less strain on your back and abdominal muscles.

Carrying

If you must carry a heavy object, carry it as close to your body as possible. For example, when carrying a bag of groceries, support it from below, carrying the weight with your lower hands and arms.

Bath Time

If you have another child to care for, you will find that bath time can be strenuous because it requires so much bending. When bending, be sure your feet are comfortably apart; bend straight from the waist, keeping your back straight. A half-kneeling and half-squatting position allows plenty of room for the growing baby and you can comfortably hand your child, the soap, and the inevitable bath toys.

You can comfortably help your child out of the bath by sitting on the side of the tub, lifting your child, standing, and then straightening your back.

CHAPTER SIX

Getting Ready

You have been preparing for birth since the onset of pregnancy by practicing good nutrition, seeing your obstetrician regularly, controlling your weight, exercising and thinking about what kind of a birth experience you would like to have.

As the time of the actual delivery draws near, you will want to start practicing some relaxation techniques to be used before, during and after surgery. You will also want to prepare your children for the arrival of a new sister or brother and set up your household for the time you will be in the hospital and also for the first few weeks or so after you return home.

EXAMINING YOUR FEELINGS

You should also begin to prepare emotionally for the cesarean. It is normal to experience some fear and dread at the thought of going into surgery as the due date draws near. The best way of coping with this is to allow yourself to feel and express your negative feelings. They may seem irrational, but you need to confront them. Many couples find it helpful to share their experiences and to have them validated by other cesarean couples. An excellent way to do this is to enroll in a cesarean childbirth class. You may also locate a cesarean support group in your community. If you continue to feel extremely anxious about having a cesarean, talking with a professional counselor may be the best thing for you to do.

Suzanne Rosno of the Cesarean Birth Council, International, suggests sitting down and writing out what you are feeling. Talk with your partner. He needs to understand and to feel needed. By sharing your innermost feelings with him, you meet both his needs and your own need to express your feelings.

Decide what you want. If being an active participant would enhance your feelings of confidence, work to maintain control in this pending cesarean birth. However, you may prefer to play a more passive role and leave the decisions entirely up to the professionals. You should not feel pressured to take a more active stance.

If you have had a prior cesarean, confronting your feelings about it is the first step toward preparing yourself emotionally for a positive cesarean experience this time. Feelings about cesarean delivery vary. There is no right or wrong viewpoint. Some women feel very good about their past experience. How you perceive the birth is related to the circumstances that surrounded it. If the experience was disturbing, you may tend to block it out because the memory is too painful to remember. Maybe you wanted to express your feelings, but no one seemed to care or was able to understand how you felt. Perhaps your feelings made other people feel uncomfortable or helpless. The advice you got from family or well-meaning friends may have been something like, "Don't dwell on it. It's behind you now" or "Just look at how beautifully formed your baby's head is. You should just be happy that you and the baby are both healthy." These comments only serve to turn off a mother's expression of feelings.

Now is the time to unbury the memories and get them out into the open so they won't have a negative influence on your perceptions of this pregnancy and birth. Some of the most common feelings we hear expressed regarding the surprise cesarean are discussed in the following sections.

Anxiety and Fear

Most couples experience some level of anxiety and fear for themselves and the baby both before and during the surgery. Some common fears are expressed thus: "I was afraid the doctors might start cutting before I was fully numb"; "I was afraid my legs wouldn't wake up after the spinal"; "I was scared that maybe I would never awake again after I was put to sleep"; "For the first time it occurred to me that my baby or I might die"; and "I was secretly afraid I might lose my wife and baby."[1]

Relief

When couples are exhausted after long hours of unsuccessful labor and discouraged because things are going wrong with the vaginal birth, they may feel relief when told that the baby must be born by cesarean. It is a relief to know that the long labor is almost over and that, regardless of the mode of delivery, the baby will soon be born.

Loss of Control

The majority of parents have less than two hours to adjust to the news that a cesarean will have to be performed, before the actual surgery begins. Two hours is not enough time to grasp what is happening and to rally your resources to face the ordeal as well as you might under different circumstances. Actually, two hours is probably the *maximum* amount of time most women get. One mother says, "Suddenly everything went wrong. I could not talk, all these things began to happen so fast. I heard all these conversations about me. I could not say anything. I was overcome with fear and pain."[2]

Suddenly the mother has no control over her body or her treatment. She may not be able to comprehend the doctor's hurried explanation. Too often, the explanations are not given or are inadequate. One woman says, "The nurse came in and looked at the monitor for a long time. She left the room without saying a word. The next time she came in, she mumbled that I was going to have a cesarean and began to shave my abdomen rapidly." Another mother remembers, "The doctor explained that the baby's heart rate went down and that he needed to operate right away. He didn't stop to explain anything."[3]

Disappointment

Many couples feel a profound sense of disappointment because they had worked and planned for a shared vaginal birth. Some individuals react with very intense feeling to the loss of this anticipated and much-valued birth experience. As one woman put it,

> John and I had practiced more than anyone else in our Lamaze class. We knew we were going to do well, and it was really important for us to be together. My water broke, but my labor never started. Finally the doctor said he would induce labor. The contractions never came and I never dilated. It ended up I had to have a cesarean. I felt it wasn't fair! Why did this have to happen to us? Another tiny girl in our Lamaze class had her baby in just three hours! I was the one with big hips, and I had to have the cesarean.[4]

And one father told us that when he learned his wife had to have a cesarean, and he was sent to the father's waiting room, he felt so angry he threw a chair against the wall.

Disorientation

Most mothers describe a feeling of "trying to put the pieces together" so they can understand what happened and why. They need to discuss in great detail the events that occurred in labor and in the cesarean delivery, to convince themselves of the reality. Sometimes they need to go over it many times, to try and rid themselves of a feeling of "incompleteness."

Depression

Feeling depressed after a surprise cesarean is a common occurrence. A woman may feel depressed after an unplanned cesarean because she is grieving, in a sense, over the loss of the birth she had desired.

This grieving state may last a few days or months. This depression is different from postpartum depression (baby blues) that many women experience after giving birth. Postpartum depression basically results from a hormonal imbalance and fatigue. (See Chapter 12 for more information on postpartum depression.)

Inadequacy

A cesarean can leave both mothers and fathers feeling inadequate. Many mothers feel inadequate and guilty. They blame themselves: "If only I had been relaxed"; "If I had practiced more"; "I am a failure because I couldn't push my baby out like other women do"; or "I let my husband down."

Some women feel as if they had been mutilated and are concerned that their husbands will find them less attractive sexually. They wonder if the cesarean will disturb their sex life.

Fathers, too, often feel inadequate. If the father was trained for natural childbirth, he knew what his role was and felt confident. Now, thrown into a cesarean situation with his wife, he feels helpless. He may feel he let his wife down because he can't be with her. How does he cope with her tears of disappointment? He feels unsure of how to help his wife recover. What should he do now? What should he say to her?

Sometimes his feelings of inadequacy continue into his fathering role. He may leave the baby's care entirely to the mother, unsure of his abilities and feeling detached.

Feeling Abnormal

Some women perceive the cesarean birth as an abnormal procedure that carries a social stigma. One mother said,

If you have a cesarean, other mothers express outright pity, and subtle and outright implications of abnormality. You feel left out, as well. It can get you down. One woman was so condescending to me that she said, "Couldn't take it, I guess." The operating room came back in my dreams regularly for two months. . . . The dreams brought back the fears and feelings of that night, a reliving of the immediate time before, and the actual emergency treatment. Perhaps it reminded me of my own mortality. The dreams come less often as time passes. They are just not as frightening. I am not left with the same internal shaky feeling. I feel guilty about my initial reaction to my son. It was so opposite from what I had expected. I looked at him and felt almost nothing. I had a hard time feeling he was even mine. At the time, I said to my husband, "How do I know that's my baby?"[5]

Detachment

The feeling of being detached from your newborn, mentioned in the preceding story, is a typical reaction following a surprise cesarean. Often a mother must work through her resentment and other negative feelings before she can experience a bond with her baby. Women often express a strong need for time to adjust to the shock of the birth experience before moving on to the task of motherhood.

Conclusion

These are just some of the reactions women have to being unprepared for a cesarean. You may be able to relate to some and not to others. You may have experienced feelings not expressed here, but if you have some feelings that bother you in regard to past cesareans or an impending one, get them out in the open. Try to resolve them so you can get on with preparing for a new birth experience.

GET PLENTY OF REST

How often during your pregnancy have you heard the warning, "Get plenty of rest"? Of all the advice commonly given, it is the most likely to be ignored. It is easier said than done, especially if you have a job or a family to take care of. Also, the importance of rest is often underestimated by most people.

Being rested is an important part of your preparation for childbirth. You should get a minimum of eight hours of sleep each night to start with, and you should also take a rest period during the daytime. In your last trimester, you should rest twice a day. Rest is more effective if your feet are elevated to at least the level of your waist or higher. This increases the circulation in your legs and pelvis. Be sure to elevate your feet if you have aching legs, swelling ankles, hemorrhoids, or varicose veins.

Another position that will be beneficial to you is to lie on your back, with a pillow under your head, and your feet elevated against the wall. You may wish to place a small pillow or folded towel under your hips to obtain a continuous angle. Rest in this position for no longer than ten to fifteen minutes several times a day.

Another excellent position to assume during your rest period is to lie on your side, with your head on a pillow. Pull your top leg toward your chest, keeping your knee comfortably bent. Support your top leg on a pillow. Be sure your bottom leg is flexed enough to reduce strain on your back. You may also wish to place a pillow under your abdomen to keep your uterus in the middle of the body, rather than shifted to right or left, which keeps body pressure off the big vein (*vena cava*) that carries blood from the legs to the heart on the right side of the spine. This is a good way to sleep toward the end of your pregnancy, when it is hard to get comfortable enough to fall asleep. This position is also good for circulation in your legs and pelvis.

One popular rest position is to lie on your back with a pillow under your head, knees slightly bent, and a pillow under your knees for support. This position is very comfortable.

As your delivery draws near, do not allow yourself to get even moderately fatigued. If you are preparing dinner or talking on the phone, sit at a tall stool, or, if possible, elevate your legs. While you are playing with your children, reading, folding clothes, or performing other household duties, sit down and elevate your feet whenever possible. Plan quiet evenings at home. Modern women tend to be very active and busy, but this is the time to pace yourself and examine your priorities.

TECHNIQUES TO REDUCE TENSION AND DISCOMFORT

Many childbirth instructors teach the following techniques to help women remain comfortable and relaxed throughout the hospital experience. Learn and practice them now for use when you feel tense or in distress during any hospital procedure such as when an intravenous is started, a blood specimen is taken, or anesthesia is administered.

Alone or in combination with medication, these techniques will also help relieve the discomfort of labor or postoperative discomfort.

Relaxation

The first technique to be learned in coping with tension and discomfort is relaxation, which is a valuable tool in the relief of pain. Relaxation is an integral part of the pain relief techniques used in Lamaze, Read, Kitzinger, and other methods of prepared childbirth that emphasize knowledge of labor and delivery, breathing, exercise and relaxation. Relaxing the abdominal muscles decreases the amount of discomfort associated with the cesarean incision and the uterine contracions that all women experience after delivery (called *afterpains*). There is a natural tendency to tense muscles in response to pain or discomfort. This tension causes more pain, and a vicious cycle is thus created. You can train yourself to respond to discomfort by relaxing instead of by tensing muscles.

Relaxation is one of the most important exercises you can practice in the weeks before surgery. Practice it twice daily several weeks prior to surgery. Two convenient times for many women are before naps and at bedtime.

Sit or lie down in a comfortable and well-supported position with your hips and knees slightly flexed (put a pillow under your knees.) Take a deep breath, contract one or two extremities (such as an arm, or an arm and a leg), and *relax the remainder of your body*. During this exercise, you or a helper should check the extremities and other parts of the body to see if they are in the proper state of relaxation or contraction. When your helper picks up your arm or leg, it should be limp and fall back on the bed when released. If you are checking yourself, your body should be limp, like a rag doll's. Hands should be open, palms up, fingers relaxed. Your mouth should be slightly open. Raise your eyebrows and let them go—this will help you relax your face. Your eyes should be lightly closed.

This exercise will teach you to relax your body. Relaxing the rest of the body while one area is contracted is difficult; there is a tendency to tense up the whole body. Learning to relax while a part of your body is contracted will help you to relax your whole body even if there is discomfort somewhere, such as in your abdomen. "Breathe in and relax as you breathe out." Say this phrase to yourself, and it will become a signal to relax. Your body will automatically respond on cue when these words are spoken. Later, during the cesarean experience, when relaxation might be helpful, your husband can pick up your arm, and check to see if your are relaxed. If you are still tense, he can say, "Take a deep breath, let go of the air, and go limp as a rag doll."

Another relaxation technique is simply to take a deep breath and blow out slowly through pursed lips.

Distraction

Distraction has been useful to mothers in reducing discomfort. The Lamaze method achieves pain relief through the use of both relaxation and distraction. The various breathing patterns and the use of a "concentration point" are forms of distraction.

Distraction may also take the form of reading an interesting magazine, playing cards, having someone give you a back rub, or working a crossword puzzle. You and your spouse may want to use such distractions while you are waiting for the time of surgery to arrive.

Another distraction technique is to focus your eyes on an object. One resourceful mother did this during the administration of the spinal anesthesia: she counted acoustical tiles in the ceiling of the operating room.

Waking Imagined Analgesia[6]

Using your imagination as a way to decrease your perception of pain is an ancient technique. Your imagination can be very powerful. Waking imagined analgesia may be defined as imagining a pleasant situation while experiencing pain or discomfort. With this technique, you *relive* all the sensations of a previous pleasant experience. Rather than just trying to *remember* the experience, try to recreate within yourself all the sensations associated with the experience. Imagine that the experience is happening again. If your imagination is active, your body will start to respond as it did when the event occurred.

There is a difference between recalling an event and actually reliving it. You may experience that difference by trying the following exercise. First, describe how you would prepare a lemon for eating, how you would hold it when you eat it, and how you would place it in your mouth to taste it. Next imagine how it tastes. Did your mouth begin to water while you were imagining the taste? If it did, you have an active imagination, and this technique will work for you.

Another example of waking imagined analgesia is recalling a ski trip. Feel the cold wind on your cheeks, hear the crunch of the snow, feel the rhythmic movements of your body as you make your way down the hill. Smell the fir trees. This example shows how you involve all your senses. When you bombard your brain with other stimuli, it becomes more difficult to perceive discomfort. Your brain will only accept so many stimuli and then "ignores" or eliminates new signals. For example, have you ever had a headache before and after an exciting movie, but not during it?

If your husband is aware that you are tense or feeling pain, he can help you by thinking of some special event in your past and by asking you to tell him in detail how you felt at that time. He should encourage you to keep your eyes open and to actually relive the experience. Verbalizing what you are imagining enhances the effect of waking imagined analgesia.

Touch

The use of touch is another effective way for your husband to distract you and help you relax. It's a natural reaction to reach out and touch someone who is hurting or nervous. For example, you can hold hands with each other. Your husband can stroke your forehead or rub your back. All this helps to relieve discomfort.

Your mind is very powerful. By using these techniques alone or in combination with pain medication, you will have a more comfortable experience.

PREPARING YOUR OLDER CHILD

For many of you, this baby will not be your first. Like most parents, one of your big concerns may be how best to prepare the child or children at home for the arrival of a new brother or sister. You are also probably concerned about your separation from the child while you are at the hospital. Your older child, up to now, has been the center of all your attention and love. You wonder, "How will he (or she) handle sharing me? How can I make his adjustment easier?" If the child is one or two years old, you feel he does not understand what a new baby is all about. You may also be worried about how you can lessen the trauma of being separated for five days. Should you let him visit you at the hospital, or will that make matters worse? These concerns and questions are frequently voiced in cesarean childbirth classes. Perhaps some thoughts and suggestions from well-known doctors, psychologists, and parents will help you prepare you child.

The baby's arrival may be a crisis in the child's life. His world has suddenly changed, and he needs help in adjusting. Dr. Fitzhugh Dodson, in his book *How to Parent,* suggests imagining that your husband comes home from work and at the dinner table announces,

"Honey, you have been such a good wife, and I love you so much that I have decided to do it again. Because I care so much for you, I'm taking a mistress. I know you're really going to like her." Or "Dear, next week Roxanne, my old girlfriend, will be joining us. Of course, I love you as much as I always have. And I will be with you on Mondays, Wednesdays, and Fridays. But on Tuesdays, Thursdays, and Saturdays, I will be with her. Sundays we will put up for grabs."[7]

Do you see any parallels in this explanation to the following one? "We love you so much and you are so very very wonderful that Daddy and I decided to have another baby, just like you. You'll love the new baby. It will be your baby, too. You'll be proud of him. And you'll always have someone to play with."

The child is, very sensibly, feeling worried rather than delighted. Sharing usually means having to give up one of his toys or getting *less* of something, like sharing an apple or a piece of candy. And even now, before the baby arrives, the child notices some changes in Mom. She is less available to him. She may be tired or resting or feeling sick. She cannot carry him anymore, and even her lap is taken up by that little baby inside her. The small child cannot articulate all this, of course, but he has a vague, uneasy feeling about it.

Most parents find that it is best to expect difficulties at first and then to be pleasantly surprised if things go smoothly. There is no way to totally take the threat away; rather, the goal is to make the transition as easy as possible for the little one at home—and for Mom and Dad, too. To be of help to a child at home, you must understand his feelings—to "walk in his shoes"—if you can.

Telling Your Child about the New Baby

Many authorities agree it is best to begin preparing your older child for the baby soon after your pregnancy is confirmed. Your pregnancy will be exciting to the whole family, and your child will become very curious and fascinated about "having babies." The level of such curiosity varies greatly, of course, depending on the age of your child. An older child will want to learn how a life begins, how a baby grows, and how it is born. It is important to encourage an atmosphere of complete openness and honesty. It is also important that you explain in correct terms; for example, say that the baby is in your uterus, not in your stomach. Otherwise your three-year-old may have an image of the baby being smothered by all the food you are eating. The maturity of the child dictates how much detail of the pregnancy and delivery are discussed. A good guideline is to answer the questions quite simply and to answer only the questions that are asked. There is no need to elaborate. Often the child wants only a one-sentence answer, and adults tend to give a dissertation on the subject.

An older child might be told that the baby is growing in the mother's uterus, that it started as an egg (or a cell) that came from a place called the *ovary* and was fertilized by something like a seed, called a *sperm,* from the father. Nine months later, when the baby is ready to be born the vagina gets bigger so that the baby can come out. A doctor usually helps the baby come out, and then the vagina gets smaller again. In Mom's case, babies are not able to be born this way. So the doctor will make a special opening on the abdomen and uterus and will take the baby out through the opening. Then the doctor will sew the opening up with a needle and thread or close it with something that looks like staples. (It might look like a zipper for a while). It will heal just like one of the cuts or scrapes that children sometimes get from playing or falling. After it is healed, the doctor will take the stitches or staples out. It doesn't hurt because the doctor gives Mommy some medicine so she won't feel the sewing or stapling (try to convey positive attitudes to your child about hospitals and doctors).

The Child Three Years and Older.   It is important to encourage an open environment where the child can feel free to talk about his (or her) feelings about the change in the family. Just as you may have ambivalent feelings about having a new child, so does your child. Convey to him that it is normal to be excited and at the same time dislike the idea of having a new baby in the house. This gives the child permission to feel and express negative feelings without feeling guilty. This creates an emotionally healthy climate for the whole family.

When telling the child about a new baby, it is helpful to give the child *realistic* expectations about newborn babies. Parents often tell a child that he will have a new brother or sister with whom to play, so the child is really surprised when he sees that newborn. One way you can help is by reading him children's books about what new babies are like and what they like to do. A visit to the nursery window of a nearby hospital or to a friend who has a young baby is also helpful. Dr. Haim Ginott gives us the following example of a helpful introduction to a future sibling:

> When Virginia, age five, found out that mother was pregnant, she reacted with great joy. She painted a picture of sunshine and roses about life with Brother. Mother did not encourage this one-

sided view of life. Instead she said, "Sometimes he will be fun, but sometimes he will be trouble. Sometimes he will cry and be a nuisance to us all. He'll wet the crib, make in his diapers, and he will stink. Mother will have to wash him, feed him, and take care of him. You may feel left out. You may feel jealous. You may even say to yourself, 'She does not love me anymore—she loves the baby.' When you feel that way, *be sure* to come and tell me, and I'll give you extra loving, so you won't have to worry. You'll know that I love you.'"[8]

Some parents may not use such an approach, being fearful that it puts ideas into a child's head. Chances are that these ideas are not new to the child. With the approach just described, you have fostered understanding and the child's freedom to say what he really thinks should he feel anger and resentment toward the baby.

The Child Under Three Years Old.   The principles of preparation that have been discussed do not apply to a child age three and under. To such children, simply say, "We are going to have a new baby in our family." This is sufficient information for a young child. Do not tell him when you first learn you are pregnant. Nine months is too long for him to wait. One month's notice is time enough.

Children at this age have difficulties conceptualizing; they can understand only things they can see and touch. They have not developed civilized ways of expressing their emotions. At this stage of growth and development, they are normally negative and defiant. They require a great deal of patience. One minute they assert their independence, and the next minute they want to be babies again. So, no matter how well you try to prepare your child for the arrival of the new baby, he is still going to display some negative behavior, which can be very stressful to you. Often it will not be the baby that is causing this behavior; it's just that the child is normally somewhat negative and defiant at this age.

Siblings and Hospital Visitation

Many hospitals are changing their policies to allow children to visit their mother while she is in the maternity ward. Often a special room is set aside for such visits. Visiting Mom in the hospital seems to help families. If your child is very young, he will probably be upset when the visit is over. There may be some crying, and the struggle of separating may actually be more disturbing to you than to your child. Nevertheless, it is best to have the child come see you. Small children need the daily reassurance that Mom is there, and seeing her helps.

A study was done at three hospitals in Cleveland to evaluate the effects of sibling visitation on one- to three-year-olds. It was found that, regardless of whether children visited mother at the hospital or not, there were more problems in daily routines at home after maternal separation. The largest increase in problems occurred in sleeping patterns. There were differences during the home reunions between children who visited and those who did not. Significantly more children who did not visit either ignored or avoided their mothers as they first entered the room and also refused their mothers' requests for hugs and kisses.[9]

Introduce your child to the new baby as soon after the birth as possible. Many misunderstandings can be cleared up right away. For example, the child will see that the baby is so tiny that it cannot be a playmate when it comes home (many children have this mistaken idea). The visit to see the newborn baby precipitates many questions by the older child. The actual homecoming becomes more casual because the child has already seen the baby as well as the mother.

Visiting Mom and the baby in the hospital helps the child at home feel more involved. Imagine how left out he might feel as he hears Daddy, grandparents, aunts, and uncles talk about the baby that he has not seen.

Some pediatricians and friends recommend that, when the new baby is brought a gift, a gift also be given to your older child. Dr. Lee Salk disagrees with this method of handling sibling rivalry:

> It can have just the opposite effect of what the parents want. I believe if you give your older child a little something each time your baby gets a gift, you only teach your older child to expect that he will get a present every time your baby gets one. This method places too much emphasis on material things, does not face up to the child's concern about the extent of your love, and is not realistic.[10]

It is better to tell your older child that new babies are often brought presents and that when he was a baby many friends who visited brought him presents. You can even get out his baby book and show him the cards and tell him what some of the presents were. Salk recommends telling your child he is not a baby any more and will not be treated like one. Your older child's real need is not for presents and new toys, but for feeling loved and having some time and attention for just the two of you. Daddy is very important, but to small children Mommy is the most important person in the world, and no one can take her place.

The best way to reassure your child is through your *actions*. Make it a high priority to give him some undivided attention without his having to demand it. Usually a child will get your attention one way or another. If he has to, he may resort to negative ways such as hitting, biting, and crying whenever the baby cries.

Nothing can change the fact that a new baby is a threat to a child's security. However, with understanding, a little knowledge, and good old-fashioned common sense, the experience can be an enriching and character-building one for your child.

Helpful Hints

The following hints can help you prepare your child for the separation and can help make life a little easier for you when you get home from the hospital. These ideas come from mothers like yourselves and, in some instances, from child psychologists. We hope that some of these suggestions will appeal to you and work out well for your family.

Involve your child in as much of the preparation for the baby as possible. Let him feel as though he's helping you as you set up the baby's room. Include him in shopping for the layette, too. Make it a fun outing for him.

Tell him how you and his daddy got ready for his birth. Explain how you felt when you were carrying him and how you looked forward to his arrival. Recall how you felt when he was born. Describe in simple terms what it is like in the hospital. Paint a pleasant picture. Children love this, and you will find it enjoyable to reflect on the happy memories of having a newly born baby.

Make arrangements early for your child's care during your stay in the hospital. Daddy and / or grandparents are favorite choices of most mothers; however, the important thing is that you have someone who is capable and loving and with whom the child feels comfortable.

Write down your child's routine and explain the way you do things, such as potty habits, bedtime routines, and the kinds of foods he eats and how he likes them prepared. Maintain the child's routine as much as possible. Arrange for his usual activities to continue, such as nursery school, play group, and visits from friends.

Plan to set out a photograph of you with your child. This is very helpful and reassuring to the three-year-old. It is not unusual for the child to talk to your picture, or to take it to bed with him along with his favorite teddy bear.

Another mother suggests leaving a taped message on a tape cassette to be played by the child whenever he wishes. You can reassure him that you are being treated fine at the hospital, that you miss him and love him. And, yes, you are coming home soon.

A problem for small children is that they have no conception of time. You or your husband might like to make a calendar with five to seven large squares on it. When you go to the hospital, place it where the child can see it. Each day you are away, Daddy can help him cross off the days.

Also, before going to the hospital you and your husband should go through your home one more time and check it for safety. The person taking care of your child is probably not accustomed to the speed or curiosity of a toddler. You may be wise to close off certain rooms by installing latches and hooks at the top of the doors. You can also purchase portable gates to block off rooms without doors, if you wish to keep the room "off limits" while you are gone.

Some people buy, address, and stamp birth announcements before they go to the hospital. When the baby is born, they fill out the information on the cards while the mother is at the hospital.

Buy ahead! You and your partner can check on what birthdays, anniversaries, and special occasions are coming up in the two months and get the gifts now. Stock up on disposable plates, napkins, diapers, and other such convenience items.

You and your husband can also prepare casseroles and frozen dinners that you can use when you lose your temporary help after coming home from the hospital. When you are preparing dinner, double the recipe and freeze half of it in a heavy-duty ziplock bag (available at the supermarket). Start doing this about a month before you are to go to the hospital, whenever it is possible. You should be able to stockpile enough frozen dinners to help you through weeks of convalescing.

CHAPTER SEVEN

Scheduling Delivery Versus Waiting for Labor

If you know in advance that you are going to have a cesarean delivery, there are two ways your cesarean delivery date may be determined. It may be scheduled by your doctor, or you can wait until you spontaneously go into labor and then have the cesarean.

In the past, doctors preferred to wait until labor began before performing a cesarean in order to guard against delivering a premature baby. Today, however, sophisticated tests exist for determining fetal maturity with little risk to the mother or baby. Consequently, many doctors prefer to schedule the day and the hour for cesarean deliveries. Interestingly, there is a new trend in this country to permit the mother to begin labor before performing a cesarean. There are some good reasons for this.

GOING INTO LABOR

The big advantage of waiting to go into labor is that, in most cases, one can rest assured that the baby has developed fully. When a cesarean is scheduled before labor begins, there is always a possibility the baby may be immature. The primary problem with an immature baby is that its lungs are not ready to handle breathing properly. The air exchange that takes place in the air sacs of the lungs with each breath

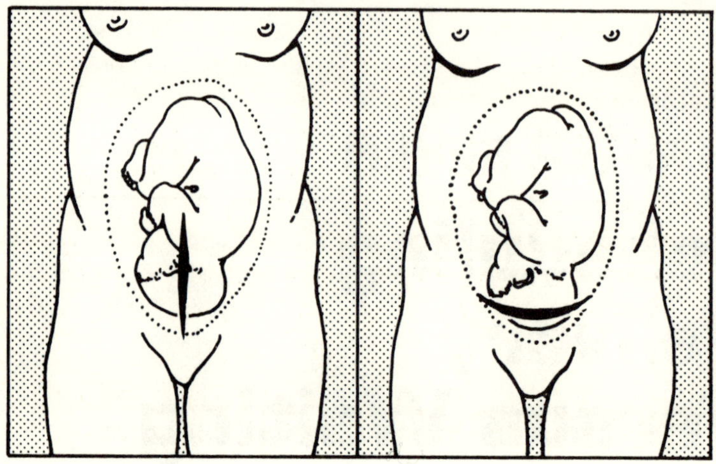

Classical incision   *Low-segment transverse incision*

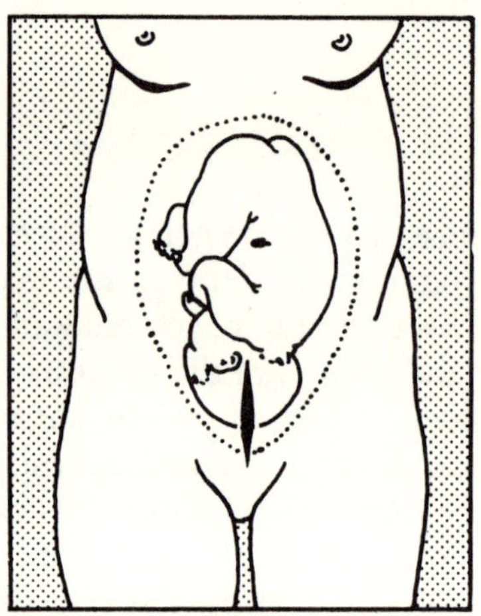

Low classical incision

is hindered. This condition is called *respiratory distress syndrome* (RDS). Another concern is that the liver may be immature, which causes jaundice. An immature nervous system also hinders the ability of the baby to keep its body warm. Thus, it is very important to determine the exact gestational age of the baby before scheduling a cesarean delivery.

A major disadvantage of going into labor is the possibility of uterine rupture. This risk is present if the mother has had a prior cesarean, particularly if the previous incision has been made in the upper uterine segment. This term refers to the incision on the uterus, not on the outer skin. Uterine rupture is unlikely to occur if the prior incision in the uterus was made across the lower third of the uterus. This is called a *low-segment incision* and will be discussed in greater detail in Chapter 16. If a cesarean mother goes into labor, the hospital should be fully equipped and prepared to handle a uterine rupture. The risk of uterine rupture is not high, but it is a potentially serious complication and requires the attention of a physician trained to handle the problem.

SCHEDULING THE CESAREAN

The advantages of scheduling the cesarean to take place before you go into labor include the following:

1. It is done at a convenient time for the doctor, the hospital, and you. Your doctor and the surgical team, including the anesthesiologist, are available at the hospital. You also can make arrangements for the care of your family while you are in the hospital, for help after you come home, and for whatever else you need to plan ahead of time.

2. You are more likely to have your choice of an anesthesiologist and/or type of anesthesia.

3. You will not have had anything to eat or drink for twelve hours before surgery, per doctor's orders. If for some reason you must have general anesthesia, the dangers of regurgitation and aspiration are greatly reduced.

4. There is less risk of uterine infection developing after surgery. The infection rate for women who have been laboring is higher. If you do not labor, your membranes stay intact and your cervix is undilated, protecting your from infection.

5. In a planned situation, everyone is more relaxed.

6. A planned cesarean provides optimal safety, as long as fetal maturity is ascertained.

DETERMINING GESTATIONAL AGE

Usually the cesarean is scheduled for one to two weeks before your due date. Your due date must be carefully calculated, and it is your doctor's obligation to procure evidence of fetal maturity. Tests such as diagnostic ultrasound and determination of the lecithin to sphingo-myelin (L/S) ratio, in the amniotic fluid, discussed below, are good indicators of fetal maturity and have made it safer to schedule cesarean deliveries on a date before the onset of labor.

The estimated date of arrival (due date) is helpful information for the doctor and can be calculated by the date of your last menstrual period. Count back three calendar months from the first day of the last menstrual period, and add seven days. This is the calendar date in the coming year when you can expect the baby to be born. Of course, some women do not have regular periods, which makes the estimated date somewhat unreliable.

The estimated due date provides, at best, a rough guess as to gestational maturity, because the length of pregnancy varies greatly. It may range from 240 days (thirty-four weeks) to 300 days (forty-two weeks) and still be entirely normal in every respect. The average duration from the time of conception is thirty-eight weeks. In view of this wide variation in the length of pregnancy, it is obviously impossible to use the "due date" as a precise indicator of the baby's age. Due dates are notoriously inaccurate!

Other indicators of fetal age include the date when the baby's heartbeat is first heard by the doctor and when the mother first feels life. These events usually take place at the end of the fifth month.

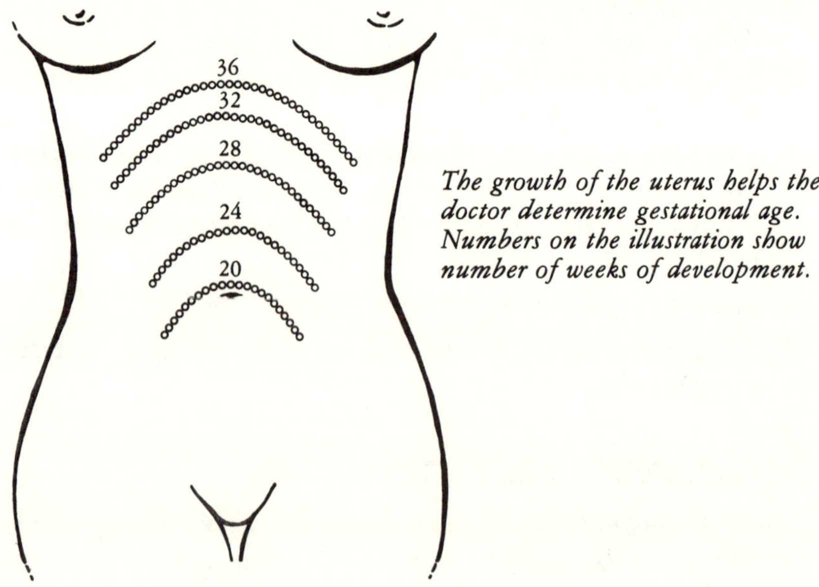

The growth of the uterus helps the doctor determine gestational age. Numbers on the illustration show number of weeks of development.

The doctor also notes and plots the growth of the uterus (height of the top of the uterus) at the time of each checkup. Again, this provides a means of estimating the growth and development of the infant.

Ultrasound

Ultrasound consists of very high frequency sound waves (2 million cycles per second), which are sent out from a quartz crystal, bounce off the baby like echoes, and return to their source. These echoes are converted into a "picture" (sonogram) of the baby. Depending on the type of equipment, the picture will be still (like a photo) or moving (like a movie).

The technology is, in a sense, akin to sonar, sound waves used to locate objects under water. It is totally different from x-rays. One reason why ultrasound was developed for obstetrical use was to find a safer way of obtaining an image of the fetus than the use of x-rays.

The primary measurement sought is that of the biparietal diameter of the baby's head, as shown in the following diagram. (Parietals are two bones forming top part of the skull.) The biparietal diameter provides an important additional piece of information in determining fetal maturity. It usually cannot be determined by ultrasound until the twelfth to fourteenth weeks. Many doctors insist that all their pregnant patients have an ultrasonic gestational age estimate in the second trimester.

Accuracy of Ultrasound Sonograms.   An early study conducted in England of the use of ultrasonic sonograms to predict delivery dates found that in only 84 percent of the cases was the delivery date accurately predicted within two weeks. Under current methodology, several sonograms are performed during the fourteen- to twenty-eight-week range, when there is maximum acceleration of growth and the greatest degree of predictability. Using these methods, gestational age has been accurately predicted, plus or minus two weeks, in 95 percent of the cases studies. The error factor of sonograms explains why many doctors do not rely on them alone to predict the gestational age of the baby.

Procedure for Ultrasound Sonograms.   The procedure for sonography is simple. You will put on a hospital gown and be asked to lie on your back on a table. Mineral oil will be smoothed on your abdomen, and an instrument like a microphone will be slowly moved back and forth across your abdomen. The sound waves generated will

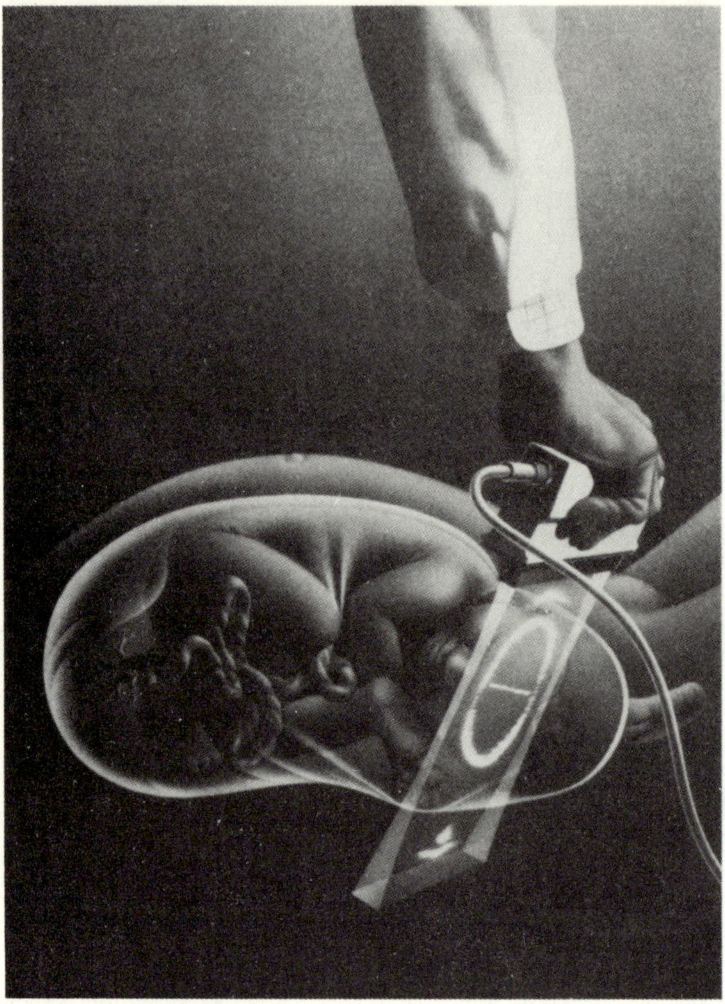

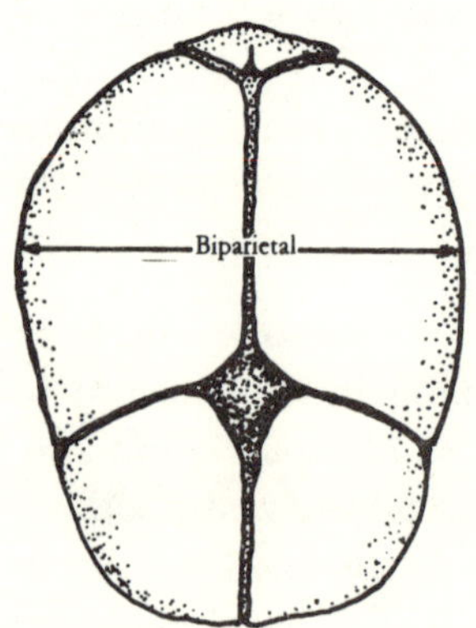

The Biparietal Diameter

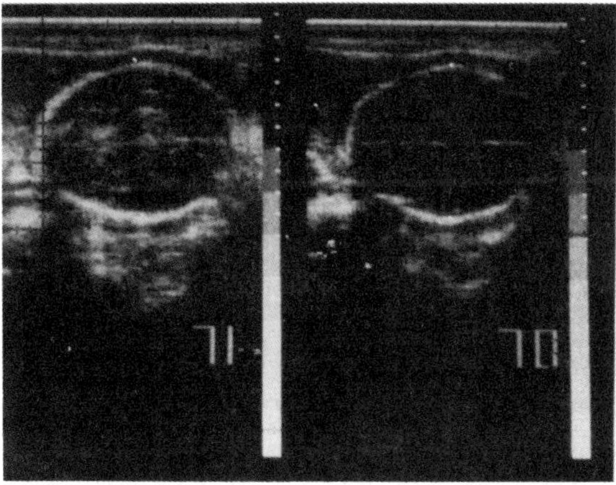

What the sonagram sees

produce the outline of the baby on a screen. The technician will take photographs of the best images on the screen for later study. These images will guide the doctor in determining whether or not the baby is mature.

The procedure is painless. Most women are excited to see the baby's heart beating or legs kicking in the image on the screen. Your husband may wish to accompany you so that he too can watch the baby. This ultrasound sonogram test may be his chance to get in on the fun.

Ultrasound Hazards. Recently there has been some concern as to whether ultrasound presents any hazards to either the infant or the mother. Ultrasonic energy interacts with tissue in several ways as yet not completely understood. However, the ultrasonic energy that would be required to produce tissue damages is of much greater magnitude than that used in obstetrics. In obstetrical use, the energy comes in short pulses, lasting about one microsecond or less, separated by relatively long intervals when the machine is "listening" for the echoes. "There have been no confirmed reports of harmful effects to the fetus produced by ultrasonic radiation at diagnostic energy levels in spite of several investigations into the matter."[1]

In considering any potential hazards of ultrasound, it is important to realize that ultrasound has been used therapeutically in physical medicine and rehabilitation for years at more energetic and lower frequency levels. No important ill effects have so far been observed from this use. In fact, ultrasound is used as a means of stimulating tissue healing.

In 1978, the FDA's Bureau of Radiological Health held meetings to discuss possible performance and safety standards for ultrasound equipment. A program of collaborative research is now being carried on to determine the extent of risk to human health posed by exposure to ultrasound in diagnostic ranges. For more information, you may write to the Federal Drug Administration, Bureau of Radiological Health, 5600 Fisher Lane, Rockville, MD 20857.

At this point in time, we do not know of any major risk in the proper diagnostic use of ultrasound. However, long-term followup studies have not been completed because the technology has not existed long enough. The risks, if any, in using ultrasound are thus unclear and appear to be clearly outweighed by the advantages.

There is no question that there are advantages of having an ultrasound sonogram. Ultrasound aids in determining the gestational age of the fetus and can be used to confirm a diagnosis of multiple gestation (twins, triplets, and so on). Ultrasound also locates the placenta. Thus, if an emergency amniocentesis must be performed, the placenta has already been located. Placenta previa can be avoided if the doctor knows where the placenta is. (Placenta previa is a condition where the placenta covers all or part of the cervix, which may make vaginal delivery impossible or cause hemorrhaging.) Although ultrasound sonography should not be routinely performed because of the expense and the slight possibility of unknown risks, in appropriate instances a woman "should not be denied the very real benefits of an ultrasound study for fear that, one day, a deleterious effect of ultrasound at diagnostic intensities will be discovered."[2]

Amniocentesis

Amniocentesis involves inserting a thin needle through the abdominal walls into the amniotic sac—the "bag of waters" within the uterus that cushions and nourishes the fetus during pregnancy—and drawing out a teaspoon of fluid to be analyzed. This procedure is generally performed for one of two reasons. Genetic testing (for abnormalities such as Down's syndrome, or mongolism) is its most common use. When done for this purpose, amniocentesis is performed early in the pregnancy to determine whether there is any abnormality in the fetus itself.

Problem pregnancies are another reason amniocentesis is done (women with diabetes, toxemia, placenta previa or abruptio, and other conditions where fetal maturity must be determined before inducing labor). In such cases, the procedure is performed relatively late in pregnancy. The test may provide the information necessary to plan the last few months of pregnancy and the type of delivery.

In a planned cesarean, some doctors routinely use amniocentesis to plan the date for surgery. They feel it is best to check the infant's lung maturity, because in their judgment the ultrasound method alone is not sufficiently accurate. They feel that any risks associated with amniocentesis are less than the risks of delivering a premature baby. Other doctors only perform this test if their data on the estimated due date, ultrasound measurements, height of the uterus, and date life is felt and the heartbeat heard do not agree in predicting a time when the baby is mature enough to be delivered.

A test is done on the amniotic fluid to determine the fluid's ratio of lecithin and sphingomyelin (L/S ratio), which indicates the baby's lung maturity. Lecithin (L) and sphingomyelin (S) are two chemicals secreted by the baby's lungs and found in the amniotic fluid. Maturation of the baby's lungs leads to changes in the amounts of these substances in the amniotic fluid. The concentration of the two chemicals is about equal until around thirty-five weeks into the gestation period, when the lecithin rises dramatically and the sphingomyelin drops slightly. The L/S ratio thus correlates directly with the degree of maturity of the baby's lungs. If the ratio is two to one or higher, it is extremely unlikely the baby will develop respiratory distress syndrome (RDS).

The L/S ratio is usually determined a couple of days before the planned delivery date. Amniocentesis in conjunction with the ultrasound sonogram test is a reliable method of determining fetal maturity.

You may wish to discuss any potential side effects of these tests with your doctor.

Procedure for Performing Amniocentesis.   A brief explanation of the amniocentesis procedure may remove some of its mystery. You may be given mild sedation to help you relax if needles make you nervous. Use of a sedative will probably be up to you. A site on your abdomen is located where the needle will avoid the fetus and be as far away from the placenta as possible when the needle is passed into the amniotic sac. The illustration shows three possible sites for taking fluid. Next the doctor will prepare the area by cleaning it thoroughly with an antiseptic and then place sterile drapes around the selected site. You will then be given a local anesthetic so you will not feel any discomfort during the procedure. Now the doctor will penetrate the

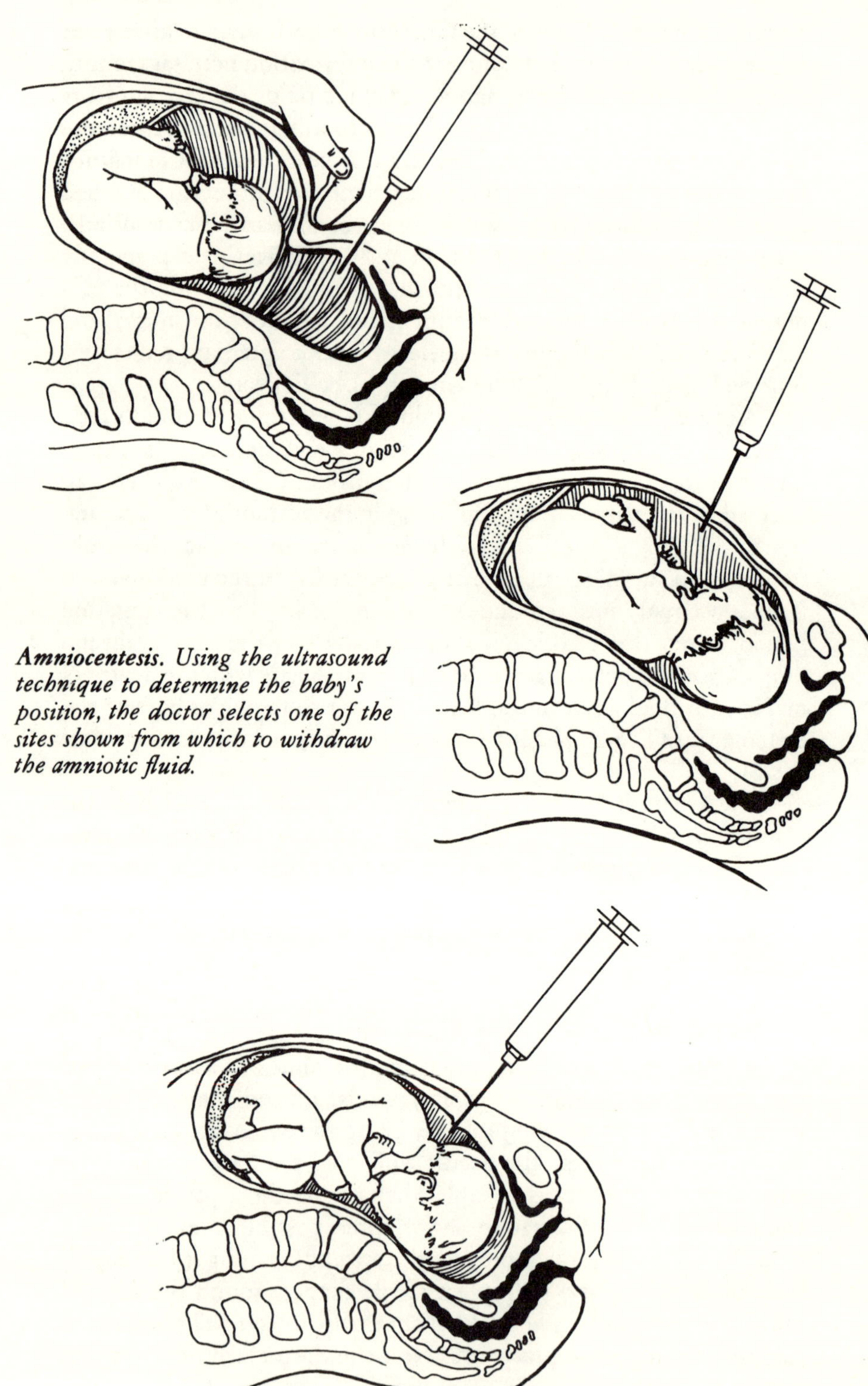

Amniocentesis. Using the ultrasound technique to determine the baby's position, the doctor selects one of the sites shown from which to withdraw the amniotic fluid.

amniotic sac gently with the needle and extract a very small amount of fluid for laboratory analysis. All this takes only about three minutes. The doctor will place a small bandage strip over the puncture site. The baby's heartbeat will be monitored at five- to fifteen-minute intervals. This is a check to make sure that there was a minimal disturbance to the baby during the procedure. After about two hours of observation, you may return to your normal activities. It will take some time for the laboratory to give you the results of your test.

PICKING THE RIGHT DATE

Concerned about the issue of ill-timed cesarean birth and the resultant RDS, the Committee on Obstetrics, Maternal and Fetal Medicine, of the American College of Obstetricians and Gynecologists, and the Committee on Fetus and Newborn of the American Academy of Pediatrics have jointly prepared and released the following statement (phrased in lay terms):

A scheduled repeat cesarean section may be performed on a patient with an uncomplicated pregnancy whose gestational age has been documented by hearing the baby's heartbeat at twenty weeks with a nonelectronic, ordinary stethoscope. This is the most reliable, safe, least expensive and noninvasive method of determining gestational age.

In situations where the baby's heartbeat was not heard at twenty weeks, other corroborative, supportive evidence of a term gestation (thirty-eight weeks) includes either of the following:

(1) Thirty-three weeks' gestation occurring after a positive pregnancy test or

(2) Biparietal diameter measurements. The first should be obtained between eighteen and twenty-six weeks' gestation. If the due date calculated by this ultrasound is within one week of the due date calculated by the menstrual date, the latter can be accepted. If, however, it does not coincide with the menstrual dates, then a second ultrasound should be obtained by the thirtieth week, no sooner than three weeks after the first ultrasound. The two measurements are then used to define gestational age.

Any one of the above criteria is acceptable evidence of a term gestation. In the absence of these criteria, the scheduled cesarean should not be done without an amniocentesis to determine lung maturity of the fetus.

In the absence of fetal lung maturity and in patients without contraindication to labor, it is a reasonable option to allow a patient to go into labor prior to repeat cesarean section.[3]

A recent study published in the *American Journal of Obstetrics and Gynecology* also addresses the issue of avoiding prematurity by correctly timing the repeat cesarean birth.[4] Although amniocentesis is a simple and relatively safe procedure, it is not entirely without risk. This study investigated the recommendation for routine amniocentesis before every scheduled cesarean. The study was done by the Harvard Medical School and the Boston Hospital for Women. During the three-year period (from January 1976 through December 1978), 1,497 repeat cesarean births were performed at the hospital.

Both pediatricians and obstetricians were concerned about the risk of RDS in scheduling repeat cesarean deliveries. Opinions vary about the use of ultrasound and amniocentesis for estimating lung maturity. Some authorities recommend that amniocentesis be performed *routinely* before scheduled delivery.

In 1974, the Boston Hospital for Women set up a policy that a cesarean would be scheduled *without resorting to amniocentesis* if the following criteria were met: (1) gestational age as determined from date of last menstrual period was confirmed by the doctor's estimate of uterine size prior to sixteen weeks, (2) the growth of the uterus remained consistent with gestational age throughout the pregnancy, (3) first fetal movement and first audible fetal heart sounds were consistent with gestational age, (4) ultrasound examination around midpregnancy (ideally between eighteen and twenty-four weeks) confirmed the gestational age, (5) the anticipated delivery was to be performed at, or after, the completion of the thirty-eighth week of pregnancy. If these criteria were not met, predelivery amniocentesis for confirmation of pulmonary maturity was strongly recommended.

Amniocentesis was considered to be advisable in 10 to 20 percent of the cases. Of the infants from the 1,497 repeat cesarean deliveries, only two developed RDS. In both cases, the recommended procedure for determining gestational age had *not* been followed. In one, early evaluation of uterine size was not documented in the records, and no ultrasound examination was performed. In the second, early examination was done and was consistent with the infant's true gestational age, but midpregnancy ultrasound was not performed, and the timing of the cesarean delivery was based on ultrasound examination performed in late pregnancy (when it tends to be less accurate).

The report concluded that amniocentesis adds little benefit for most women in whom the duration of pregnancy by menstrual history is confirmed by examination before sixteen weeks and by ultrasound between eighteen and twenty-four weeks, whose uterine growth and dates for first movements and first audible heartbeat are appropriate, and for whom scheduled cesarean delivery is planned after completion of the thirty-eighth week. The researchers noted that "Our findings support the view that confirmation of pulmonary maturity by amniocentesis should be reserved for those patients in whom assessment of the above-mentioned parameters is either incomplete or inconsistent."[5]

SIGNS OF LABOR

After you have had the tests to determine fetal maturity and the doctor has set a delivery date, the baby may still decide to come early. This does happen occasionally, so you should be able to recognize the signs of labor and know what to do.

"Lightening" or "engagement" usually occurs two to three weeks before labor starts with your first baby. Women often say, "The baby is dropping." The baby's head, if the baby is head down, usually settles down into the opening of the pelvis. You will know when the baby is "engaged" in the pelvis because you will be able to breathe more comfortably. You will not feel as much pressure under your rib cage. You may feel, instead, pressure behind your pubic bone, a need to urinate more frequently, and more difficulty walking. If you have already had a baby, engagement may occur simultaneously with the beginning of labor.

Another sign that labor may occur soon is increased discharge of vaginal mucus, which often takes place a few days before labor begins. The small mucus plug blocking the cervix breaks loose. This discharge is called "pink" or "bloody show" because it is often blood-tinged. It is usually a sign of early labor but may occur as early as two weeks before labor begins.

Often women lose two or three pounds shortly before the onset of labor. Other women experience the "nesting instinct," a spurt of energy—a need to clean house in readiness for the baby. Resist this urge. Rest instead!

Before labor, you may have feelings similar to those experienced just before a menstrual period. You may feel some cramps, pressure in your rectum, and a need to urinate frequently.

Toward the end of pregnancy, the muscles of the uterus are getting ready for labor. From time to time, you will feel them tighten and then relax. These contractions usually cause little discomfort. You may not even feel them. Sometimes they become stronger in late pregnancy, and you may have to stop what you are doing for a moment during each contraction. Some women experience "false labor," which consists of strong, irregular contractions that come and go for several hours. They are quite normal, so do not worry about them. Sometimes they are difficult to tell apart from real labor, so it is best to *call the doctor when you feel any strong contractions late in pregnancy.*

Labor contractions generally are regular and become stronger and stronger as time progresses. However, some women's labor contractions are not regular.

A gush or trickle of fluid from the vagina means that the bag of waters (amniotic sac) has broken. This is a sign of pending labor and should be reported to the doctor without delay. Sometimes the amniotic sac remains intact until the end of labor, so do not wait for this to happen before calling the doctor if you are experiencing other signs of labor. If any of these signs of labor appear, call your doctor immediately. He (or she) will probably have you go to the hospital for an examination in order to confirm that labor has begun.

PART III
The Baby Arrives

Indications for a Cesarean

Most women have no idea before beginning labor that they will require a cesarean section, except in repeat cesareans. The obstetrician makes the decision if during labor it becomes apparent that the delivery is not progressing as it should. He (or she) exercises his professional judgment based on his knowledge and experience in order to achieve the dual goals of a safe birth and a healthy baby.

Some indications for a cesarean delivery are absolute. In such cases, there is no reasonable alternative, because labor and vaginal delivery would endanger the mother or child. In other instances, the decision is more difficult. A vaginal delivery may be possible but not as safe as a cesarean delivery. The obstetrician must assess the situation and make a decision. A cesarean section is considered relatively low risk surgery, but it is also major surgery, so the doctors will consider carefully before deciding to perform the operation.

Unless abdominal delivery must be performed as quickly as possible, your doctor will have time to explain your condition and his decision to you and the father. But the ideal time for learning about the various reasons for performing cesareans is now, not during a labor contraction while you are trying to cope with the news that the doctor thinks he should take the baby by cesarean.

CEPHALOPELVIC DISPROPORTION

Cephalopelvic disproportion is the most common reason for a primary cesarean section. The prefix *cephalo-* means head. Celphalopelvic disproportion means there is a disproportion between the size of the baby's head and the size or shape of the mother's pelvis that prevents the baby's head from moving down the birth canal. A failure of labor to progress alerts the doctor to the possibility of your having cephalo-pelvic disproportion.

Your doctor can confirm his suspicions by using an x-ray and ultrasound sonogram. The x-ray will provide the doctor with information about the size and shape of the mother's pelvis. The sonogram will show the size and shape of the baby's head. Armed with this information, the doctor is in a position to know if a cesarean is appropriate.

ABNORMAL POSITIONS

Ideally, when labor begins, the baby will have assumed a head-first fetal position called the *vertex presentation* (*presentation* is a term applied to the manner of the baby presenting itself to the examining finger at the mouth of the uterus) in which he will slide down the birth canal with his stomach facing his mother's spine. When the baby is in the vertex position, the *smallest* dimension of the baby's head is the first part of the baby moving against the cervix with each contraction. This dimension is later the first part of the baby to move through the birth canal. During labor, the baby's head acts as a sort of wedge, helping to dilate the opening of the uterus known as the cervix. The baby's head is constructed in such a way that it can change shape as it passes through the birth canal. The baby's head is "molded" to accommodate the shape of the mother's pelvis. Molding is able to take place because the bones which make up the baby's skull are not fused together at the time of the baby's birth: (Later, at about one year of age, these bones of the skull will fuse together.) The elonga-

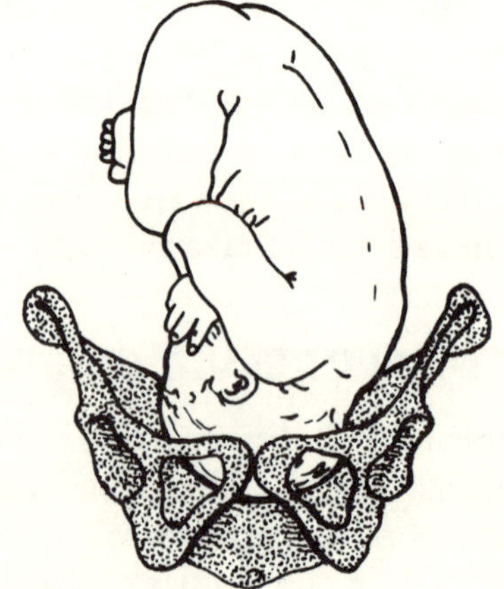

Vertex Presentation (head down; this is the ideal position as labor begins)

tion of the baby's head produced during the birth process may persist for a period of days; but don't worry, it isn't permanent.

If at the onset of labor, the baby assumes an abnormal position, such as breech, transverse lie, or posterior position, labor and delivery may be more difficult or, in some instances, even impossible.

Breech

The best known type of abnormal position is the "breech presentation," in which the buttocks or feet of the baby instead of the head are presented at the uterine outlet. There are three basic varieties of breech presentation. In the *frank breech*, the baby's legs are straight up with the feet near the baby's head. In the *complete breech* presentation, the baby's legs are crossed Indian style. In a rare breech position called *footling*, one or two feet come down the birth canal first.

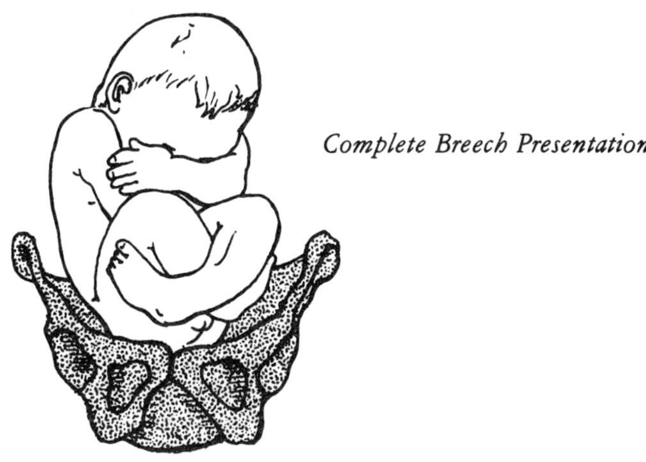

Complete Breech Presentation

At some point in your pregnancy, your baby had probably been in a breech position because the baby continually moves around in the uterus well into the third trimester. As the baby becomes larger, room to move around freely in the uterus diminishes and the baby usually will eventually get into the head-down position. During the last few weeks of pregnancy, the baby's position becomes stabilized. It can, however, change positions up until the time labor begins.

The doctor becomes aware of the breech presentation when examining the mother's abdomen. A breech presentation will be confirmed by a vaginal examination in which the doctor or nurse feels the soft, irregular buttocks, genitalia, or a foot, rather than the smooth, hard dome of the baby's head.

Because there are many risks associated with delivering a breech baby vaginally, the current medical practice by the majority of doctors is to deliver all breeches by cesarean. This trend has contributed by 10 to 15 percent to the rising cesarean birth rate.[1] Deepening concern over the rising cesarean rate has caused medical and lay persons to carefully consider the issues surrounding the automatic delivery of a breech baby by surgical means.

What are the Risks of Breech Vaginal Delivery?   Breech presentation may result in a long labor that does not produce complete dilation of the cervix. The baby's head at birth is the largest part of his anatomy. If the head can be delivered vaginally, then the rest of the body will slip out also. When a baby is in the breech position, a smaller buttocks, foot or shoulder comes first and the rest of the baby's body may be pushed through an *incompletely* dilated cervix by the strength of the uterine contractions. The larger, following head of the baby may not be able to pass through an incompletely dilated cervix, resulting in the head being trapped inside the uterus. To make things worse, the cervix may close around the baby's neck after the shoulders have passed through.

The baby may be pulled out with the aid of Piper forceps (special, long forceps designed to be used for delivering the heads of breech babies) but this may cause tearing of the cervix. It is believed to be better to incise the cervix, but this is very difficult to do when the body of the baby is in the way. As the doctor struggles to deliver the baby's head, the baby's oxygen supply is cut off by the pressure placed on the cord as it is caught between the baby's body and the mother's bony pelvis. Babies may suffer permanent brain damage and even die if the baby's oxygen supply is cut off for too long.

The baby's head, since it exits last, has no time to be molded to accommodate the shape of the mother's pelvis so it may get "hung up" in her pelvis as well as at the cervix.

Besides the problems already mentioned, there are other risks associated with breech births. There is a greater possibility of prolapse of the umbilical cord, which occurs when the cord comes down the birth canal before anything else. With prolapse, there is a possibility that the cord will become compressed, interrupting the baby's oxygen supply.

Fractures, dislocations and nerve damage are more common with breech deliveries than with other deliveries.

These problems occur in only a small percentage of breech deliveries, but it is impossible to accurately predict ahead of time which babies will be adversely affected. However, there are some factors which are felt to favor the outcome of a breech delivery and there are some doctors who will attempt a vaginal breech delivery in certain sit-uations. The National Institute of Health Task Force on Cesarean Childbirth recommends that vaginal breech delivery should be con-sidered an acceptable manner of delivery if a) the baby's anticipated weight is less than eight pounds; b) the mother has a normal pelvis in shape and size; c) the baby is in frank breech position; d) the head is not hyperextended (with its chin up and its head tilted back); and e) the delivery is conducted by a doctor with experience in vaginal breech delivery.[2]

Even these guidelines have some problems. For instance, it isn't possible to accurately predict a baby's weight ahead of time and there is no guarantee that a baby under eight pounds will have a small head. Some babies, regardless of weight, just have large heads.

The Changing Breech Position. Some doctors and midwives will attempt to turn a breech baby by manipulating the outside of the mother's adbomen. This is called "external version." It is not advisa-ble because the baby usually resumes its breech position after having been turned. More importantly, it is dangerous to the mother and baby. The baby can be endangered by the cord becoming entangled or the placenta separating from the uterine wall. The danger to the mother is that of uterine rupture.

It is wise to await the onset of labor if your doctor's practice is to deliver all breech babies by cesarean. There is always the chance that the baby may spontaneously turn to the vertex (head-down) position and you may proceed to labor and deliver vaginally without any risk to your baby.

Vaginal Delivery with a Breech. If your doctor plans to allow you to attempt a vaginal breech delivery, he probably will discuss the potential dangers with you ahead of time and should involve you and your mate in making the decision. You may wish to get a second opinion. Each case should be judged individually.

The doctor will probably x-ray your pelvis ahead of labor to check its size and shape. Ultrasound measurements of the baby's head and determination of the baby's position may also be obtained (see page 67). Knowledge of your pelvis and the baby's head size will ena-ble the doctor to see if the baby's head can fit through your pelvis. (One of the problems with breech delivery is that a disproportion be-

Abnormal Positions

Abnormal Positions.
*This is the same
baby, with its head
in varying positions.
Note how this posi-
tion change alters
the width of the part
coming first through
the birth canal.*

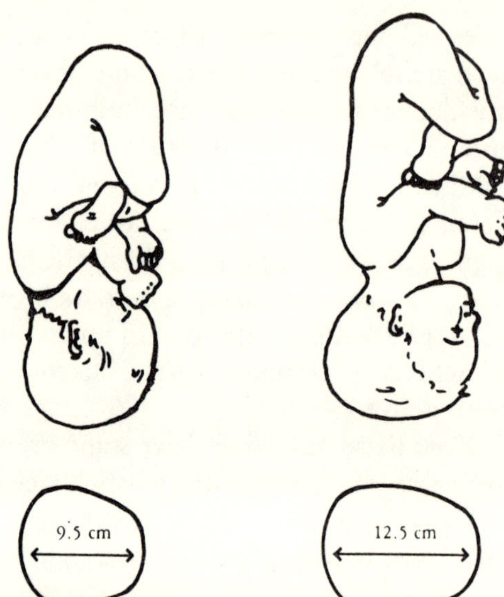

*This is the measurement of the
baby's head in vertex position
(smallest dimension coming
first down birth canal).*

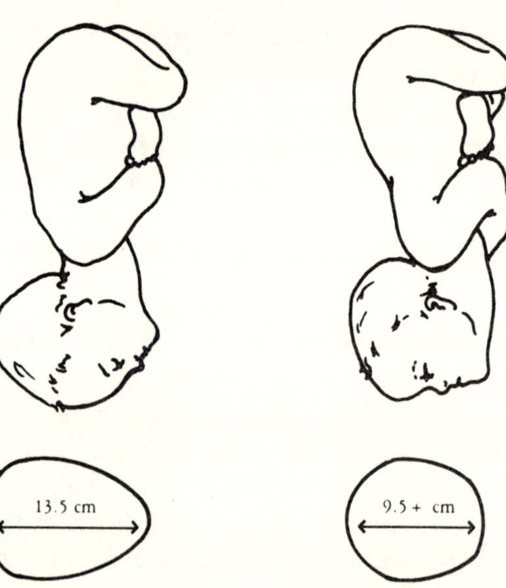

*This shows measurement
when baby is in brow
presentation.*

*This the the measurement
of the baby's head in face
presentation.*

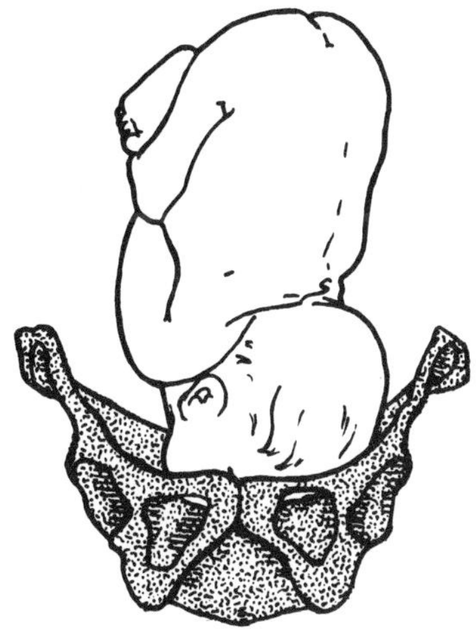

Face Presentation

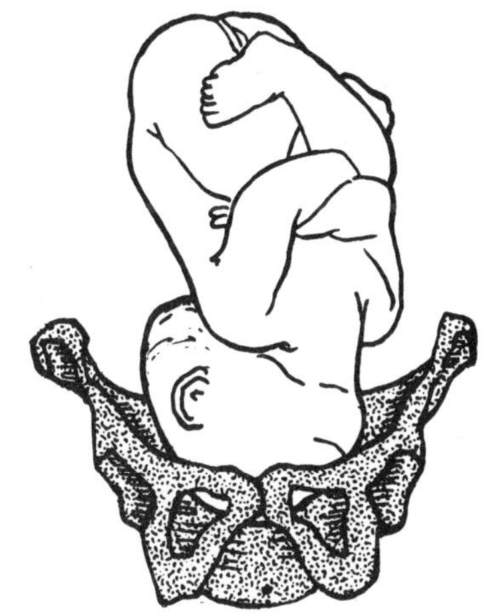

Posterior Presentation

tween the baby's head and your pelvis size may not be known until after the baby's body is born.)

The doctor will also try to estimate the baby's weight. The baby's estimated weight should be between 5 to 8 pounds. Babies under 5 pounds have a greater risk in a breech vaginal birth. Because they are small, it is more likely that their bodies will be delivered with an incompletely dilated cervix, and then the larger head can't get out. Also, their brains are more vulnerable to both trauma and lack of oxygen. Moreover, there is a greater chance of umbilical cord accidents.

A breech delivery is considered a "high risk" situation and will be closely monitored with a fetal monitor. If you undergo a vaginal breech delivery, you may sense tension among the nurses and the doctor. You may even go through labor and delivery in the cesarean room with an anesthesiologist in attendance so that a cesarean can be done immediately if necessary.

If during labor there is any fetal distress, or your labor does not progress (you don't continue to dilate), the doctor will probably do a cesarean. As mentioned earlier, the labor may be slowed or hindered because of the buttocks rather than the head coming first. Fetal distress can be caused by a lengthy, difficult labor that stresses the baby or by compression of the umbilical cord.

Gravity may be used to help the baby make its way down the birth canal. Sitting is an ideal labor position. The best is to sit straight up with your knees out at your sides and the soles of your feet together.

Piper forceps are often used to gently keep the baby's head flexed down on its chest during its delivery.

The delivery completed, you may be startled by the baby's swollen genitals or black and blue buttocks. This is due to the pressure of labor and delivery, but goes away quickly and does not cause permanent damage.

Another presentation which can cause problems occurs when the baby arrives face first or brow first. This presents the largest diameter of the baby's head. If the baby's head is large and the mother's pelvis small, a cesarean delivery may be necessary.

One absolute indication for a cesarean is when the baby is positioned horizontally to the ground rather than vertically with the head down. This is called *transverse lie*. It is the most dangerous position, because vaginal birth of a living infant is impossible in such cases unless the baby is extremely small.

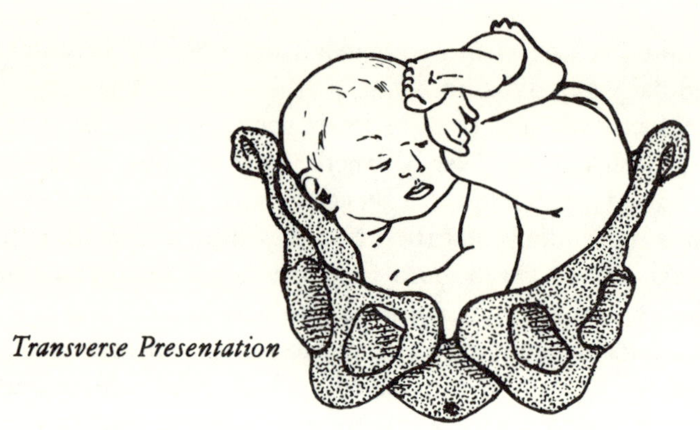

Transverse Presentation

FETAL DISTRESS

An increasingly frequent indication for a cesarean is fetal distress. The use of a fetal monitor facilitates earlier and more accurate detection of fetal distress during labor.

The fetal monitor can detect if the umbilical cord is prolapsed (enters the birth canal before the baby does), which may threaten the baby's life. With a fetal monitor, the obstetrical team can simultaneously record the baby's heartbeat and the mother's contractions. If the baby's heartbeat undergoes certain changes in relation to the mother's contractions, this indicates that the baby is not getting enough oxygen. Such a condition is referred to as *fetal distress*. When fetal distress is indicated, the doctor may elect a cesarean delivery rather than a lengthy labor and vaginal delivery to ensure the birth of a completely healthy baby.

There is some controversy regarding the use of the fetal monitor. Critics say it limits the woman's mobility and thus may interfere with the labor process, because walking and certain positions may help labor. Also, the monitor may be incorrectly interpreted. If fetal distress is identified, ideally the diagnosis is verified by a fetal scalp blood test.

Fetal distress is almost always caused by a decrease in flow of oxygen-rich blood to the baby. This usually causes the pH (measure of acidity and alkalinity) of the baby's blood to be lowered. Too low a pH means the baby's health is in jeopardy and must be delivered immediately, perhaps by cesarean.

The sample of baby's blood is taken by inserting a special cone-shaped speculum (an instrument the doctor uses to gently dilate the vagina and visualize the uterine cervix, as when doing a Pap smear) into the vagina, which is moved up against the baby's head (if the baby is in the head-down position), and making a tiny prick. A few drops of blood are taken, and its concentration of oxygen and carbon dioxide and its pH are tested.

Some hospitals do not have the capability to do this test quickly. This should be a consideration in selecting the hospital for your delivery.

The fetal monitor is a much more reliable tool if used in conjunction with fetal scalp sampling. Mothers who will be experiencing labor would be wise to discuss the fetal monitor in more detail with their doctors.

PLACENTA PREVIA

Normally the placenta is attached high up in the uterus, but in the condition called *placenta previa* it is attached in the lower third of the uterus. It may partially or entirely cover the opening of the uterus to the birth canal.

If the placenta completely covers the opening of the uterus, a cesarean delivery is absolutely necessary because the baby's passage is blocked. When the placenta partially blocks the baby's exit, a safe vaginal delivery may still be possible, depending on the degree of blockage and bleeding.

Painless vaginal bleeding is the main symptom of placenta previa. The bleeding generally occurs after the seventh month. It may begin as spotting and increase, or it may start with profuse bleeding.

The bleeding is caused by the separation of the placenta from the uterine wall as a result of changes that take place in the uterus during the later months.

If the bleeding is slight, the doctor may observe the mother carefully, allowing the baby to approach full gestational age before scheduling a cesarean. If there is profuse bleeding, surgery will be done at once.

Fortunately, placenta previa is not a common condition, but it must always be regarded as probable cause for a cesarean section.

PLACENTA ABRUPTIO

In the conditon called *placenta abruptio,* a normally located placenta detaches from the uterine wall prematurely. This is characterized by bleeding and abdominal pain. When this happens, the blood circulation between mother and infant is compromised and your doctor will perform a cesarean.

INEFFECTIVE LABOR

Sometimes, despite many hours of labor, the cervix fails to dilate. There are many reasons for this failure of labor to progress. Perhaps the baby's head refused to move through the pelvis because the head is too large or is in an unusual position. Perhaps the uterine contractions are not sufficiently strong. This condition is known as *uterine inertia,* and its cause is unknown. It is thought that it may be due to the age of the mother or to the excessive or premature use of pain medication. Labor lasting over twenty-four hours without significant progress may be a reason for a cesarean delivery.

HERPES SIMPLEX VIRUS II

Herpes Simples Virus II is the second most prevalent venereal disease in the United States today. It manifests itself with lesions on the vaginal lining or the cervix. These lesions are fluid-filled blisters that can appear on any part of the body, but usually appear around the genital area. (Herpes Simples Virus II should not be confused with Herpes Simplex I, which only causes cold sores and is not dangerous to the baby.) Herpes II is transmitted to the baby about 50 percent of the time during a vaginal birth as he passes through the infected birth canal. If the baby develops Herpes II, he will die or suffer severe nerve and/or eye damage. A woman who has ever had Herpes II is thus a candidate for a cesarean and must have a thorough examination by her doctor as the delivery date approaches, to make sure the virus is not active. Unfortunately, an inactive Herpes II virus tends to become active when a woman is pregnant. Also, an inactive virus tends to become active, causing an outbreak of lesions, when a woman is tense, suffering from a vitamin B deficiency, or is in her menstrual cycle. Pregnant women with Herpes II should eat nutritious foods regularly, get plenty of sleep, and wear loose-fitting undergarments to prevent an active flareup at delivery time.

If a woman has active Herpes II lesions in the vagina or cervix at the time of labor, a cesarean must be performed to protect the baby before the membranes rupture or within four hours of the rupture (the membranes hold the "bag of waters"). Therefore, if you have ever had, or do have, active Herpes II and your bag of waters ruptures, get to the hospital immediately.

OTHER INDICATIONS

Other indications for a cesarean delivery are maternal diabetes, toxemia, or cardiac disease. In the case of toxemia (eclampsia), the pregnancy often must be ended as quickly as possible to save the mother's life (the pregnancy is causing the toxic condition). And for women with severe diabetes or heart disease, the stress of long labor might endanger their lives as well as their babies' lives.

REPEAT CESAREAN BIRTHS

Most obstetricians in this country believe that "Once a cesarean, always a cesarean." The concern is that strong labor contractions may lead to uterine rupture, endangering mother and child.

Some doctors may disagree with this policy and will attempt vaginal birth under certain circumstances. Factors considered are the reason for the previous cesarean, the size of the baby and your pelvis, the type of previous incision, the hospital facilities, and the availability of anesthesia, blood banking, and operating room personnel. (See Chapter 16 for a more extensive discussion.)

The reasons for having a cesarean are many. Some indications are absolute, and others require the considered judgment of your obstetrician.

CHAPTER NINE

Hospital Admissions and Preparation for Surgery

You may know from the outset of your pregnancy that you will be having a cesarean, or you may find out only minutes before the birth. If you are having a scheduled repeat cesarean, you know ahead of time what day surgery is set for, and you may want to preadmit to the hospital.

BEFORE ADMISSION

At many hospitals, you have the option of getting some necessary admission tests and paperwork completed before the day you are admitted for surgery. This is called *preadmission*. A urinalysis, blood tests, and sometimes an EKG (electrocardiogram) can be done up to forty-eight hours before surgery.

The following tests are routine and must be performed for any surgery patients. The urinalysis will test for urinary tract infections. A blood count is done to verify that you are not anemic and to test for any bodily infection. A blood specimen will be used to type and match several units of blood that will be available in the event that you should need a transfusion.

ADMISSION

If you have not been preadmitted, when you arrive at the hospital you will go to the admission office. There you will be asked to register and fill out various hospital forms. You will need to present your insurance forms at that time, so have them ready. When these tasks are completed, a plastic identification bracelet will be placed on your wrist.

You will then go to the maternity department. A nurse will greet you and show you to your room. You will be asked to change into a hospital gown and get into bed. A nurse will check your pulse, temperature, blood pressure, and respiration. The baby's heartbeat will also be checked.

The father can be present throughout the admission procedure but later, when you are being prepped, he may be asked to step out for a while.

PREPPING

Prepping encompasses all the preparation for surgery. The nurses will remove your jewelry and lock it up. If you wish to wear your wedding ring or a religious medal, you will be permitted to do so (your wedding ring will be taped on your finger so it cannot slip off). If you are wearing nail polish, it will also be removed. The reason for this is that most anesthesiologists want to be able to assess your nails for color during surgery, because nail color shows the level of oxygen in your blood. (You may as well cancel that manicure!)

Do not be surprised when a nurse appears with a razor, soap, and water and announces that she is going to shave you from just below your breasts to midthigh. This "prep" is necessary to ensure a clean area at and around the incision, because bacteria cling even to the nearly invisible hairs. An area much larger than the incision is routinely prepared in this fashion. The nurses are experienced in prepping, so don't be concerned about getting an "early incision."

If you are opposed to this total prep, tell your doctor about it ahead of time, and he may arrange for you to get a partial prep. Some doctors do not have the abdomen shaved in preparation for cesarean surgery; there is some evidence that it may not be necessary.

OTHER PROCEDURES

It should be mentioned that the doctor may have ordered an enema for you in order to empty your intestines. If he has, you are going to be feeling very clean, inside and out, by this time. The enema prevents constipation from pain medication and inactivity; straining to have a bowel movement when one has an abdominal incision is to be avoided.

Shortly before you are taken to the operating room area, a nurse will probably give you a preoperative injection. This will probably not be a sedative and does not harm the baby. Its function is to dry up the secretions normally produced in your mouth, throat, and respiratory passages. It also increases the rate of your heartbeat. Both these effects are very beneficial to you during surgery and will cause you no discomfort. If general anesthesia becomes necessary (if the regional anesthesia is incomplete), it is easier for the anesthesiologist to keep the patient's airways free of mucus if mouth secretions are dried up. A side effect of anesthesia may be a drop in heart rate and/or blood pressure, so this drug is given to reduce the likelihood of such effects. Also, some doctors prescribe an antacid to neutralize your stomach. The antacid reduces stomach acid so that any vomiting that might occur will not result in aspiration pneumonia if the anesthesia must become general. See Chapter 10 for a more complete discussion of these drugs.

THE ANESTHESIOLOGIST VISITS

Sometime before surgery, the anesthesiologist will visit you to discuss your medical history and the type of anesthesia he (or she) will want to administer. It is good for the father to be present for this exchange of information. He may also have some questions he would like to talk over with the anesthesiologist. (Anesthesia is discussed in greater detail in the next chapter.)

SCHEDULING SURGERY

The sequence of the procedure we have discussed will vary somewhat depending on whether you are preadmitted and when you are scheduled for surgery. Also, practices vary among different hospitals. Usually cesareans are scheduled for early morning (around 7 A.M.) or about noon. Depending on the doctor's schedule and other variables, you may or may not be able to choose the hour of your surgery.

If you are scheduled for early morning surgery, you will check into the hospital the afternoon or evening before surgery so that necessary preparations can be made. You will have the option of receiving a sleeping pill at the hospital. When the nurse wakes you in the morning, you know that your surgery will take place within a couple of hours, so you have less time to wait and "watch the clock" than you would if you were not scheduled until noon. (By noon, the doctors are often running late, so you may not go to surgery precisely at the appointed time.)

Also, if you are at the hospital the night before surgery, the nurses can make sure you will be N.P.O. (that is the hospital abbreviation of the Latin phrase *nihil per os,* meaning "nothing by mouth") from midnight on. The nurses can also see that you are well hydrated (have drunk lots of fluid) and get a good dinner before you go "N.P.O." Your husband would also be well advised to eat well and be hydrated so he won't get sick or feel faint during the surgery, if he plans to be present.

Other mothers feel they sleep better at home (hospitals can be noisy). They may want to spend the night before surgery with their families. These mothers would prefer to have surgery around noon and enter the hospital that morning. No matter what your preference, it is important to get a good night's sleep and try to relax.

The father's love and support will be a comfort to you during the hours preceding surgery. Turn your thoughts to the miracle that is about to take place—the baby you have carried for nine months will soon be in your arms to love.

CHAPTER TEN
Anesthesia

The material on anesthesia was not the last subject researched, nor was it to be the last chapter in the book, but it was the last chapter written. The reason was that Marty and I could not agree on how much material to include on this topic. Marty, the nurse and childbirth instructor, wanted to include more detail than I felt necessary. I, a cesarean mother and the world's biggest coward, would have been happy to merely allude to anesthesia in some other chapter, if at all. I had many arguments against Marty's approach. "Come on," I said, "We're not medical students, we're mothers to be: All you will do is scare the mothers to death with all that technical information. It's unproductive."

But Marty has worked with cesarean mothers in a teaching capacity for a long time, and she explained to me what she had learned from the mothers and fathers in her classes. She told me, "The subject of anesthesia arouses various levels of fear in just about everybody. Women have different ways of coping with fear. Some women, like yourself, cope better by not dwelling too much on the unpleasant aspects of the delivery and by thinking about happier things related to the birth experience. They would rather leave the worry of the anesthesia up to the professionals. This is fine for these women. It works best for them." That was me, all right. I remember when the anesthesiologist came to my hospital bed the night before surgery, as is customary, to discuss the anesthesia and tell me about possible side effects of the drug, I resented having to hear it all. I had to suppress a wild urge to hurl my water glass at him as he left the room, all the while knowing in my heart he was a good doctor and just doing a difficult job the best he could. When the time came to have the anesthesia administered, I would think hard about something else. I always planned well ahead of time what I would think about, in case I panicked at the last minute and couldn't think of anything. (This, by the way, is a legitimate "relaxation technique" taught in many childbirth classes as a means of coping with pain and tension. We have discussed these techniques in Chapter 6.) Distracting myself helped a great deal, but I still really hated the procedure. It isn't very painful—I've had more pain from a toothache, a stubbed toe, or a bee sting. It's the fear—the fear of needles—the fear of the unknown and the sense of losing control over my bodily functions.

As if reading my thoughts, Marty went on to say, "It's not the pain so much, it's the fear. The fear of the unknown is very strong in some people. Most women in my classes cope best with the fear by learning all they can about anesthesia. They want to know what is happening to their bodies. They want to know what they might feel, the various side effects, and how to make the most of the situation. They also need enough information to make an informed decision about their anesthesia preference. Many of these same women will want to make an appointment to talk to the anesthesiologist well ahead of the delivery date. The more they know, the more comfortable they feel. We need to provide them with the information to meet these various needs."

That argument had a familiar ring. That was what our book was about all along. I was ready to write. We agreed to provide all the information we could on anesthesia for those interested in learning about it, and to encourage a meaningful dialogue between mother and anesthesiologist, if that is your desire. It certainly is your right. Anesthesia is an important part of your cesarean experience.

No two people go through life with identical experiences. This is as true of your anesthetic experience during your cesarean as it is of anything else in life. Your experience will be unique. Some generalizations can be made about what you may expect, but some events unique to you will occur.

The anesthesiologist will try to visit you the night before your cesarean delivery to discuss your anesthesia preference, answer your questions, and choose the anesthetic he feels is best for you and your baby.

The choice of an anesthesia will depend on a number of factors, including your condition, the reason for your cesarean, your obstetrician's preference, your anesthesiologist's preference, *your* preference, and the practice in your hospital. When choosing which drugs and anesthetics to use, the comfort and safety of the mother and the baby are considered.

Regardless of the type of anesthesia you will receive, an intravenous drip will be started in your arm to provide you with fluids and nourishment and to allow the anesthesiologist to give you intravenous medication on a moment's notice just by inserting the appropriate drug into the intravenous tubing.

GENERAL ANESTHESIA

If you are given general anesthesia, you will be unconscious during surgery. General anesthesia is used in any sort of emergency situation, because every minute counts and this is the fastest means of administering anesthesia. In a "surprise" cesarean delivery, when you are unprepared, exhausted from labor, and scared, you may feel very happy to be put out and wake up as a new mother. Even in a planned cesarean, many women prefer to be put to sleep for surgery. There is virtually no situation in which general anesthesia cannot be given, from a medical point of view. General anesthesia is thus usually selected when there is severe fetal distress and/or maternal bleeding with conditions such as placenta previa, placenta abruptio, and prolapsed cord (see Chapter 8, on indications for a cesarean delivery). General anesthesia is the best method when time is of the essence.

Risks of General Anesthesia

The major risk associated with general anesthesia is that, as you lose consciousness, you also lose control over most body functions and reflexes. Of most concern is the loss of the swallowing and gag reflexes that keep your windpipe clear. Without these protective mechanisms, whatever is in your stomach may roll up into your mouth and then back down your windpipe and into the lungs, where it can cause a very serious pneumonia. (Don't you wish you had a water glass to throw at me?) This is called *aspiration pneumonia* and is especially a risk in unplanned cesareans, because most such patients have recently eaten when they go into labor. Once labor begins, digestion more or less stops. Anything that was in your stomach is just going to sit there until the digestive process resumes.

With a planned cesarean, you will not be allowed to eat or drink anything after midnight, so your stomach will be empty. Also, to minimize the risk of aspiration pneumonia you may be given an antacid an hour or so before surgery to neutralize the acid in your stomach. Stomach acid can burn the lungs. Many anesthesiologists prescribe a shot to dry and temporarily shut off the acid secretion in your stomach. The only effect you will feel is an incredibly dry mouth. Usually a soft, flexible tube is inserted into your windpipe. Before you panic, let me hasten to add that this is done after you have been put to sleep. You won't feel a thing. The danger of aspiration is thus limited to the few moments between the time you go to sleep and the tube is in place.

A second disadvantage of general anesthesia is that it limits the amount of time in which to deliver the baby, so the obstetrician is racing the clock. Usually the baby is delivered within ten minutes from the start of the anesthesia, and most studies indicate that if the baby is delivered within ten minutes, the baby will not be unduly sleepy or depressed. But, if the surgeon works much beyond fifteen minutes, then the baby becomes markedly sleepy from the anesthetic continually going into the mother. After birth, as the baby takes a few breaths and exhales the gas-type anesthetic, he will quickly wake up. A long-range test has not been devised to see if general anesthesia under these circumstances has any effect on the child. Because the effects of being sleepy the first minute of birth from anesthetic agents are not known, anesthesiologists try to avoid this situation on the theory that it is simply better to have an alert, crying baby.

To prevent the baby from getting too much general anesthetic, general anesthesia is induced at the very last moment. So, if you wonder why you are lying there and the nurse is washing off your abbomen, putting the sterile sheets on, and clanging instruments around while you are getting nervous—this is by design. The anesthesiologist waits until everything is ready and the surgeon is literally standing there with scalpel in hand before you are put to sleep. It minimizes the time from the start of the anesthesia to the delivery of the baby, so the baby receives a minimal amount of anesthetic.

About 15 to 20 percent of cesarean patients retain some memory of the surgery. This occurs because, with general anesthesia, the anesthesiologist deliberately gives you the lightest anesthesia possible while still keeping you from feeling pain or being awake. Certain things seem to penetrate the lightly anesthetized mind, so some women have some memory or recall of surgery. They usually do not remember pain but they may remember things that were very important to them (such as the doctor saying, "It's a girl!") or something worrisome (such as, "She's bleeding a lot").

Another factor to consider is your recovery from general anesthesia. Usually you will receive Pentothal, or a similar drug, intravenously to start the anesthesia. Once you are asleep, the anesthesiologist switches over to a gas type of anesthetic and may add some intravenous narcotic or something such as Valium. As a result, there is a substantial quantity of drugs in your body. How long does it take for your body to excrete these drugs from your system?

The amount of time varies from person to person. Some women feel groggy for only a few hours after surgery. Other women report that it took them several days to a week before they felt really awake, alert, and back to their normal, unanesthetized selves again. Most women excrete almost all the anesthetic after twenty-four hours. The time depends on the individual's body chemistry and how it metabolizes drugs. If you have had general anesthesia before, you probably have some idea how your body reacts. It will probably respond similarly this time.

After you awake from general anesthesia, you will probably feel pain from the incision almost immediately. The onset of the pain will be more sudden than the gradual onset that occurs with the regional anesthesias. Pain medication will be ordered for you, so ask the nurse for it.

During the immediate recovery period some women become nauseated by the gas anesthetics and/or from having had their organs moved around during surgery. The nurse can give you something to prevent or relieve nausea while you are in the recovery room.

REGIONAL ANESTHESIA

From a personal viewpoint, the big advantage of regional anesthesia is that you are awake for the birth of your baby and can perhaps share this event with someone else close to you—usually the father.

From a medical viewpoint, a big advantage is that your reflexes, particularly your protective airway reflexes, are operative. You are in control of your breathing. If you should throw up some food, you can turn your head and cough. It is safer if your own body is in control of these functions. If you are unconscious, the anesthesiologist must control these functions.

Another big advantage is that the baby receives little or no anesthesia because you are receiving a relatively small amount of a local anesthetic in a part in your back that is relatively closed off from the rest of your body. The anesthetic attaches itself to the nerve roots and numbs them, so there is very little, if any, free anesthetic in your bloodstream and crossing the placenta to the baby. Your nerves are numb, but the baby is awake and vigorous.

With regional anesthesia, the surgeon has plenty of time in

which to deliver the baby. It does not make a difference in the baby's condition whether he (or she) comes out in five minutes or twenty minutes. This is a particularly significant factor in a second or third cesarean, which often takes a little longer because the surgeon is cutting through an old, scarred incision. The surgeon must go more slowly. With regional anesthesia, surgeons feel that they can take their time, and they are more relaxed because they know the baby is not getting sleepier and sleepier with each minute.

Risks of Using Regional Anesthesia

The main risk of regional anesthesia is the potential drop in blood pressure. Beside numbing the nerves that carry pain, pressure, and touch messages to the brain, regional anesthesia numbs the nerves that control blood vessels. The blood vessels lose their tone, becoming relaxed or dilated, and do not move the blood along as well as normally. This condition can lead to a drop in blood pressure. Generally, the blood pressure does not fall so low that it endangers the mother, but it can compromise the blood flow to the placenta. This can be serious, because the blood is carrying oxygen to the baby. Precautions are taken to avoid a drop in blood pressure. If it should happen, it's reassuring to know that you will be given drugs intravenously to raise the blood pressure back up to normal. When the mother's blood pressure is low already, as occurs with bleeding, regional anesthesia is not advised.

There are also other situations when regional anesthesia is not indicated. As mentioned earlier, if it is important to deliver the baby within minutes regional anesthesia takes too long to administer, so general anesthesia would be used. Also, if you have a skin infection on your back or an internal infection spreading throughout your system, using regional anesthesia risks bringing the infection, via the needle, to the nerves.

If you have back problems, from mild back pain to extensive back surgery, regional anesthesia would probably not be considered. Anesthesiologists do not like to risk aggravating already existing back problems. Also, some back conditions and prior surgery make it anatomically difficult or impossible to administer regional anesthesia.

Differences Between Spinal and Epidural Anesthesias

Spinal and epidural anesthetics are administered in a similar manner and give similar effects. There are some advantages to each. We asked Dr. Sidney Helperin, of the University of California at Los

Angeles, to explain to us the differences between spinal and epidural anesthesias. We also asked him to tell us something about the procedure of administering the drug, and what one might expect to feel. He provided us the information that follows.

If you are to receive an epidural or spinal anesthetic, you will be asked to lie on your side and curl up like the curve of a rainbow. The baby will be in the way of your knees, but the more you curl up the more you will open the spaces between your vertebrae and the easier it will be for the anesthesiologist to place the needle correctly. Lying still and not pulling away also makes the anesthesiologist's job easier. The nurse will help you get into position and will help steady you. (Sometimes, however, you will be asked to sit up for the administration of the anesthetic.)

Before giving you the anesthetic, the anesthesiologist will wash your back with a cold antiseptic solution. Then you will feel him probing with his fingers for anatomical landmarks (the space between the vertebrae). He usually explains to you step by step what he is doing before he does it, so there are no surprises. If he doesn't keep you informed, feel free to request that he do so. After cleaning your back, he will make a numb spot with a tiny needle so that you will not feel the epidural or spinal needle. He may also deposit some local anesthetic just under the skin and along the path to be taken by the spinal or epidural needle. As he injects this local anesthetic, you may feel a slight stinging sensation. Both the epidural needle and the spinal needle travel along the same path. The epidural needle stops short of the dura, which is a touch membrane that helps contain the spinal fluid. *Dura* means "tough" or "durable," and *epidural* means "on the dura," so the epidural is closer to your skin.

For a spinal, the needle is inserted *through* the dura into the space containing the spinal fluid. When the needle (spinal or epidural) is in place, the anesthetic solution is injected. Only a small volume of anesthetic solution is used for spinal anesthesia, because the spinal is more central and anesthesia blocks the nerve roots closer to the spinal cord. A larger volume is used for epidural anesthesia.

You will be asked to lie on your back as soon as the anesthetic has been administered. The spinal anesthetic will make you numb almost instantly. The epidural anesthetic will take fifteen or twenty minutes to have its full effect. You may or may not feel a pins-and-needles or tingling sensation in your legs. You may have a sense of warmth in your legs. You probably will not be able to move your legs (the motor nerves, as well as the pain nerves, are blocked). Within an hour or so after the completion of the cesarean, normal sensations and movement begin to return.

After the anesthetic has been administered and you are on your back, the nurse will wash your abdomen with an antiseptic solution. You will probably feel her do this. *When the obstetrician performs the cesarean, you won't feel any pain, but you will feel pushing, pulling, and pressing.* In some cases, it is possible for some sensation of pain to get through, usually of a mild nature. The anesthesiologist can help you through such episodes by distraction, the use of relaxation techniques, or by administering additional drugs.

You may experience sensations of light-headedness, nausea, vomiting, feeling faint, or difficulty in breathing. Simply tell the anesthesiologist what you feel, and he can take care of it.

To make sure the baby gets enough oxygen, the anesthesiologist usually gives you oxygen with a plastic mask or a nasal cannula (a soft plastic tube inserted about 1/4 inch into the nostrils). He may remove this after the birth of the baby.

The baby is born five to ten minutes after the cesarean begins. Once the baby is born, the anesthesiologist feels no hesitation about giving you more sedation if you need it.

Usually the operation and the anesthesia proceed smoothly and routinely. If minor problems occur, they are taken care of as they happen. However, occasionally a condition develops that warrants the utmost attention of the anesthesiologist, the obstetrician, and all others concerned. Should such a situation arise while the husband is in the room, his presence may be a distraction and may divert necessary attention from the mother and baby. In these circumstances, the father, if present, will be asked to leave, and should do so without a moment's hesitation.

With both spinal and epidural anesthesia, numbness occasionally extends a little higher than the breasts. When this occurs, the patient may not *feel* herself breathing even though she *is* breathing. This can be very frightening, especially if she is not prepared for this possible but rare occurrence. You can be assured that the anesthesiologist is watching your breathing at all times. The regional anesthesia wears off in reverse order, so your sense of breathing will come back first and you will be able to feel your chest moving up and down again.

An extreme form of this condition occurs when a spinal block goes so high that it numbs you all the way up to your neck and above. When it does go this high, a mask is used to give you extra oxygen and help your breathing. When the block goes this high, you are still breathing but require assistance. Usually you become sleepy, so you are not alert and frightened. One woman who experienced this relates, "I wanted to say that my chest felt numb but the next thing I knew I was asleep." This "high spinal" only occurs with spinal, not epidural anesthesia. It certainly does not happen very often but is a potential problem. However, it can be managed quite safely.

Spinal Headache

"Spinal headache"—the sound of it alone is enough to make you want to ask for an epidural. However, although it is true that nobody ever got an "epidural headache," the chance of getting spinal headache is also rare.

In spinal anesthesia, the needle penetrates the dura to enter what is called the *spinal space,* which is filled with cerebral spinal fluid. It is thought that the tiny puncture causes a few people to get spinal headache (mild to severe) about the second day after it has been administered. Although the possibility of getting spinal headache does exist, with the small needles that are now being used it is very unlikely. The headache, if it occurs, usually doesn't last more than two or three days. Mothers who have headaches find they are more comfortable if they lie flat and drink lots of fluids. Pain medication is also helpful.

The Recovery Period

We asked Dr. Susan Sheridan of the University of California at Los Angeles, if there were any differences between recovering from spinal anesthesia and recovering from epidural. She explained,

> Depending upon which drug is used as the anesthetic agent, the numbness can last from an hour and a half to three or four hours. Their effects gradually diminish, and all sensation and movement come back. Just as the spinal anesthesia has a rapid onset, so it terminates more abruptly than an epidural. You may feel totally numb and cannot move. . . . Fifteen minutes later it's all worn off, and all of a sudden your stomach hurts where the incision was.
>
> With epidural anesthesia, the effects wear off more gradually. Usually movement comes back first, and you can see your legs moving but you cannot really feel them yet. Pressure comes back next. Pain, is the last sensation to come back. So women tend to recover nicely in the recovery room because they are awake and alert, they are moving their legs, and yet they are still comfortable. As sensation returns gradually and some incisional discomfort begins to be felt, they can ask for pain medication,

which probably will be needed for at least the first twenty-four hours.[1]

Because the regional anesthesias leave you awake and free from the pain that will later come when the effects of the anesthesia have worn off, recovery time is a great time for you and your husband to get acquainted with and enjoy the newborn. If someone doesn't bring the baby, ask for him (or her). If the baby's condition is stable and hospital policy permits, you should be able to have your baby for a while. This is a peak time for sharing.

MAKING A CHOICE

If you are going to have a cesarean, what type of anesthesia would be best for you? Beside the advantages and disadvantages of the anesthesias already presented here, there are other factors to consider. These include the hospital, the anesthesiologist and his or her training. In most states, nurse anesthetists may not give regional anesthesia. So, if you are delivering in a small hospital that just has a nurse anesthetist, you are going to have to go to sleep; unfortunately, there is no choice. Most larger hospitals have anesthesiologists (M.D.'s) who are allowed to administer regional anesthesia.

Epidural anesthesia is technically more difficult to administer than a spinal block. Many anesthesiologists who only do obstetric anesthesia part time may therefore lack the expertise for administering epidurals. If that is the case, spinal anesthesia is definitely better. Because he uses it all the time in general surgery, the anesthesiologist will be proficient at the spinal anesthesia technique. Properly performed spinal anesthesia is very satisfactory.

Whichever choice you make, your anesthetic experience is an integral part of the cesarean procedure. Your anesthesiologist will use his training and experience to the best of his ability to ensure that you have a minimum of discomfort and that you and your baby will have a maximum of safety.

CHAPTER ELEVEN

The Cesarean Delivery

In the hours before delivery, you may become tense as the pending surgery becomes a reality. This is an exciting time. After all the waiting and speculating about the mysterious little person within you, the time has come for the secret to be revealed, as you welcome a new family member. Try to keep your thoughts away from the surgery itself and concentrate on the miracle about to take place and on the new person about to enter the family.

FINAL PREPARATIONS FOR SURGERY

When the doctors are ready for you to be moved to the operating room, you will be lifted onto a gurney (a stretcher on wheels) and wheeled to the operating table. The exact order of events that follow will vary according to your hospital's routine.

When you are shifted onto the operating table, an intravenous (IV) solution will be started in your arm. The purpose of the IV is to give you medications, replace body fluids, and replace blood if necessary. Because drugs can be administered directly into the bloodstream through the IV, they will take effect within seconds. An IV should not be uncomfortable after the initial needle prick, so if it hurts let the doctor or nurse know.

A blood pressure cuff will be placed on one of your arms so the anesthesiologist can monitor your blood pressure throughout surgery.

A cardiac monitor often is used to monitor your heartbeat. If so, small electrodes will be placed on your chest. The doctor uses these devices to check your vital signs (the signs that indicate vitality, such as blood pressure and heart rate).

ANESTHESIA

Anesthesia is discussed in greater detail in the preceding chapter; here we will just review the basic procedure.

If you are having spinal or epidural anesthesia, you will be asked to turn on your side and curl up into a ball with your chin tucked into your chest and your knees pulled up to your chest. This is quite a feat when you are nine months pregnant!

For some women, *anticipating* a spinal or epidural may be the most frightening part of the cesarean birth. Relaxation techniques will be very helpful at this time. If you have taken any Lamaze or Bradley childbirth classes, you are already familiar with some techniques. If not, refer to the discussion of relaxation techniques in Chapter 6 of this book. Some women find it helpful to establish eye contact with someone in the room or to hold a nurse's hand while the spinal is administered.

The anesthesiologist will tell you everything he is going to do before he does it. He will paint your back with an antiseptic solution and then numb a small area of the back with a drug similar to novocaine. This may sting for a minute. The doctor will then probe with his fingers to find the correct spot to administer the spinal or epidural anesthesia. He will inject a single dose of anesthetic. Most women say it feels "just like having a regular shot," but women who have a spinal while in labor may find the experience painful, because their tolerance for pain is very low.

After the spinal or epidural is given, you will be asked to turn over on your back as quickly as possible. The anesthetic, if spinal, begins to take effect almost immediately. Your legs will feel warm and tingly and then numb. A common side effect of spinal or epidural anesthesia is a feeling of nausea, which passes quickly. If it doesn't, tell the doctor. Medication or slow, deep breaths of oxygen will relieve it.

CATHETERIZATION

A catheter (tube) will be inserted into your bladder to keep it empty and flat during surgery. The catheter also enables the nurse to check your kidney function immediately after surgery. Another benefit to having a catheter is that you will not have to use a bedpan during the immediate postoperative period. The catheter will usually remain in place for twenty-four to forty-eight hours.

SCRUBBING AND DRAPING

For both regional and general anesthesia, an anesthesia screen will be placed at your shoulders. Its primary purpose is to keep you from breathing on the sterile area. It also prevents you from seeing the surgery, because it is about eighteen inches high. If the father is present (see Chapter 15), he will be seated next to the mother, and his visual field will also be restricted. If the father wishes to witness the birth of his baby, he may be invited to stand up and look over the top of the screen moments before the baby is born.

ADMINISTERING OXYGEN

An oxygen mask may be placed over your mouth and nose. This is done to increase the amount of oxygen going to the baby. Sometimes little plastic prongs about three-quarters of an inch long, connected to tubes, are placed in your nostrils instead of the mask.

YOU ARE READY

You have now undergone all the preparatory procedures, and in this sense you are "ready" for surgery to begin. If you have had regional anesthesia, you are also "ready" in another sense—you will feel a sharpening of your senses and an increased alertness. One mother relates, "I felt almost superhuman. All I was lacking was my Wonder Woman costume in maternity size." This may be an exaggeration, but these feelings of readiness are mediated by the sympathetic nervous system to prepare your body for optimal functioning during a time of stress. You will be aware of, and a part of, everything going on around you, so in a very real way you will feel you are participating in the birth of your baby.

You may be surprised at the number of people in the surgical suite. In addition to the doctors who will perform the surgery, there is the pediatrician, anesthesiologist, nursery nurse, scrub nurse, and circulating nurse. If your husband is present, he will be seated near your head. He will not be allowed to move anywhere unless he is escorted by a nurse.

THE SURGERY

If you are having a repeat cesarean, the incision will be made at the site of the old cesarean scar. The old scar tissue is removed, and the doctor incises one layer of tissue at a time. He controls any bleeding by tying off larger blood vessels with sutures and electrocautery (an electric current is used to coagulate the small blood vessels). His assistant keeps the surgical site free of blood by dabbing it with a gauze "sponge."

You may overhear some conversation between the doctors that you will not understand. For example, "Give me an Alice." They are not rooting for a girl baby to be delivered. That is the name for a commonly used surgical instrument. If you hear things you wonder about, you may ask the anesthesiologist.

When the layers have been cut, the doctor can see the uterus, which is a purple color. He will make a three- or four-inch incision in the wall of the uterus. Sometimes the bag of waters is cut simultaneously, and there is a gush of straw-colored amniotic fluid. If the bag of waters is intact, the surgeon will make a small opening and suction out the amniotic fluid. You will hear the suction catheter, and this will tell you the birth is imminent.

Your baby will be born about five to ten minutes after the surgery begins. Repairing the various abdominal layers after the baby has been born takes an additional thirty to forty-five minutes.

The obstetrician will pull the baby's head out first. The exception to this is the breech baby, who will arrive in this world bottom first. The mucus will be suctioned from the baby's nose and mouth. This will only take seconds, but it may seem like an eternity to you and the father, who are waiting anxiously for the doctor to pull out the rest of the body so you can see if you have a boy or a girl. Now the baby is pulled out. He gives a lusty cry that proclaims his arrival. The delivery room echoes with cries of "Oh, it's a boy" or "It's a beautiful baby girl," or "Look how big he is!" or "She's got your black hair."

After nine months of waiting and yearning to get your hands on your baby, it seems unfair that the first contact the baby has in the outside world is with the doctors and not with you. Unfortunately, there are some procedures that must take precedence.

First the umbilical cord must be clamped. The pediatrician will then take the baby over to a special heated crib to check the baby's breathing. (Hopefully not before he has held the baby up for you to get a glimpse of your seconds-old baby, all wet and covered with the vernix (a creamy substance that protects the baby's skin while the baby is floating in the amniotic fluid). It is an important moment and a memory that should not be denied you.) Ideally, the crib is placed close to the mother so she can watch. It is normal for a newborn to breathe in an incoordinated fashion—bursts of rapid, increasingly deeper breaths follow a period of gasps, chokes, sneezes, and no perceptible breathing. Although this breathing pattern can be frightening to new parents, it causes the pediatrician no alarm.

He may suction the baby some more. He may even place a tiny plastic tube down the baby's nose or throat to suction some straw-colored mucus from the baby's stomach. Frequently, he will give the baby extra oxygen to ensure an adequate supply.

The pediatrician checks the infant's heartbeat, respirations and cry, reflexes, muscle tone, and skin color. Then he gives it an Apgar score: Each of the factors just mentioned are evaluated at one- and five-minute intervals and given a score of 0, 1, or 2. These scores are added together to get a total score, 10 being the maximum. This is an indication of the baby's condition.

BABY GOES TO THE NURSERY

The baby will shortly be taken to the nursery, where the nurses rinse the blood and vernix from the infant, wash him with a medicated soap to avoid infection, and inject him with vitamin K to prevent internal bleeding.

The infant is weighed and measured, and this information is recorded. The infant will be footprinted. Most states require by law that a drop of silver nitrate be put in the baby's eyes, to prevent ophthalmia neonatorum, an infection of the baby's eyes if the mother has undiagnosed gonorrhea.

Some hospitals require that cesarean babies be observed in an isolette (incubator) for twelve to twenty-four hours after birth. Here they can be left undressed so they are more easily observed; their body temperature is maintained at normal levels by the warming element in the isolette. However, more and more often hospitals are allowing the mother and baby to spend much time together the first day. Finding out this kind of information early in your pregnancy may influence your choice in selecting a hospital and pediatrician.

COMPLETION OF SURGERY

Now that your baby has been born, your interest in the surgery has waned, but you still have to be sewn up. As the stitching begins, synthetic oxytocin (a hormone) will be added to your IV fluid, causing your uterus to contract to the size of a grapefruit. Each layer of tissue that has been cut must be carefully sewn, and this may take approximately thirty minutes. How you will feel during suturing varies and cannot be predicted ahead of time. Some mothers have arranged with the anesthesiologist to be put to sleep while they are being sewn up, in which case the father, if present in surgery, may go to the nursery with the baby. Other mothers plan to stay awake. If the latter is your preference, tell the anesthesiologist when, and in what way, you feel uncomfortable should you feel any pain during the suturing. He will help you through any rough times by administering additional drugs. If the father is with you, he will be helpful in distracting you from the surgery and helping you to relax.

The final skin closure, which will be removed before you go home, may be regular stitches, dissolvable stitches, or something like metal staples. A sterile dressing is usually placed over the incision. You will be rolled gently onto a gurney or bed and brought to the room where you will recover.

THE RECOVERY ROOM

You will spend the next two or three hours in the recovery room, where you will be carefully monitored by a nurse who is trained in caring for patients who have just undergone surgery. In some hospitals, this specially equipped room will be a recovery room used only for new mothers. If you are in this type of room, the father and baby may be allowed to stay with you. However, in other hospitals the recovery room is for all surgical patients, and you may find yourself being recovered with the old gentleman who has just had a gallstone operation and the girl who has had an appendectomy. In this type of room, the father and baby probably will not be allowed to visit.

Your state of alertness will range from groggy to wide awake, depending on what drugs you received during surgery. If you find yourself shaking and your teeth chattering for a while, do not be alarmed, because this is a common occurrence.

You will remain in the recovery area until your condition has stabilized and the effects of the anesthesia have worn off. If you had a spinal or epidural, this means until you are able to move your legs. During this time, the nurse will be checking your blood pressure, pulse, vaginal flow, and urine bag to make certain your body is functioning normally. She will monitor your IV. She will press on your abdomen to see if your uterus is contracted. If it feels "soft," she will massage your abdomen, helping your uterus to contract, which prevents hemorrhaging after the delivery. This contraction may cause an intermittent cramping sensation that can be painful but that does not last long. It is very important to keep the uterus in a contracted state.

The nurse will ask you to wiggle your toes and bend your knees. If you cannot do this at first, you will be able to do so later as the anesthetic gradually wears off. As sensation begins to come back to your legs, they may feel oddly uncomfortable and "prickly," but not painful. At your incision, you may begin to feel a burning sensation. If it becomes painful, the nurse may give you an injection to ease the pain if you are adequately recovered from the anesthetic.

You will be wise to start your abdominal tightening exercises in the recovery room. Your reaction to that statement is probably "You've got to be kidding!" It will take self-discipline, but the abbominal exercises should be started within one hour after delivery and should be done four or five times each hour while you are awake for the next five days. This will prevent the development of gas pains, which otherwise may cause you much pain in the days to come. The exercise is done as follows: Hold your incision with both hands, take a deep breath, and exhale. Take another deep breath, hold it to a slow count of five and exhale. Finish with a cleansing breath, just in and out. You may not be comfortable the first time you attempt this but do not give up. It gets easier. *Your incision will not come apart.* You may not use that as an excuse! It is good for you to finish this exercise with a deep, strong cough from your abdomen. There is a discussion on coughing in Chapter 12.

When you are ready to leave the recovery room and to be moved to your own room in the maternity unit, you may pass by the nursery. This is an opportunity to see the big attraction through the nursery window or maybe even to hold the little character who is stealing the show.

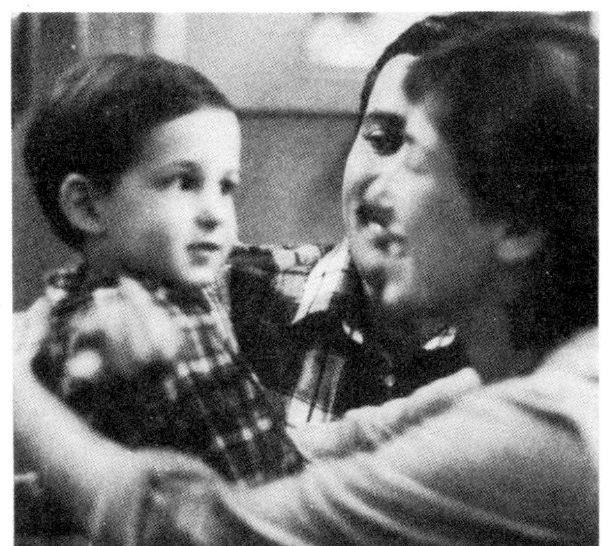

Barbara and Jack are expecting their second child, in a father-attended cesarean birth. Their first child was born by a surprise cesarean.

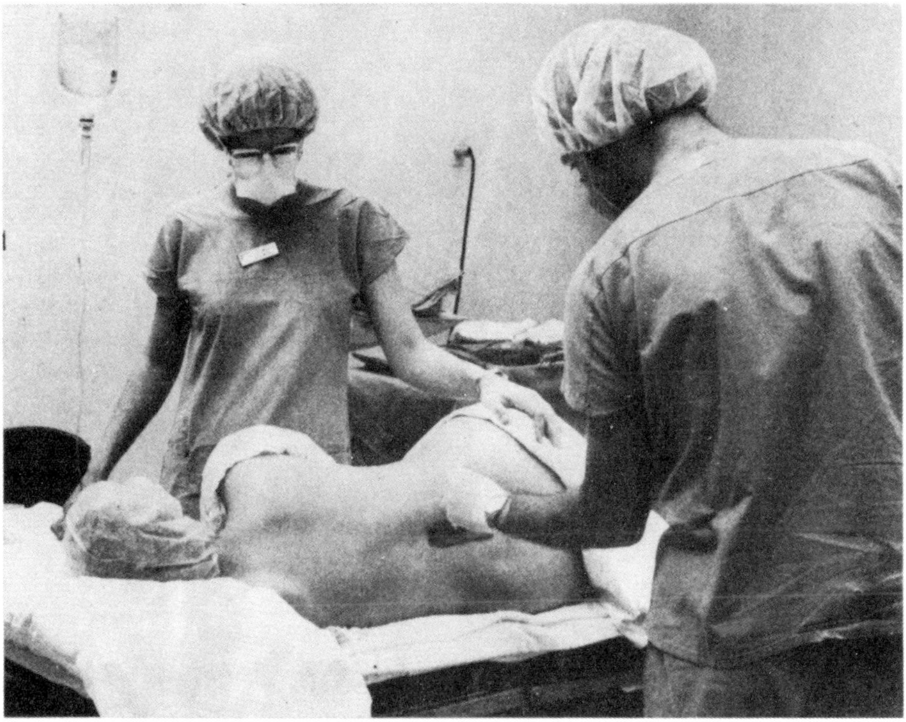

Barbara is being prepared for surgery. A blood pressure cuff is placed on her arm, and cardiac leads are placed on her chest. Barbara is told to pull her knees up to her chest. The anesthesiologist probes to find the space between the vertebrae where the anesthetic will be administered. He numbs the area and cleans it.

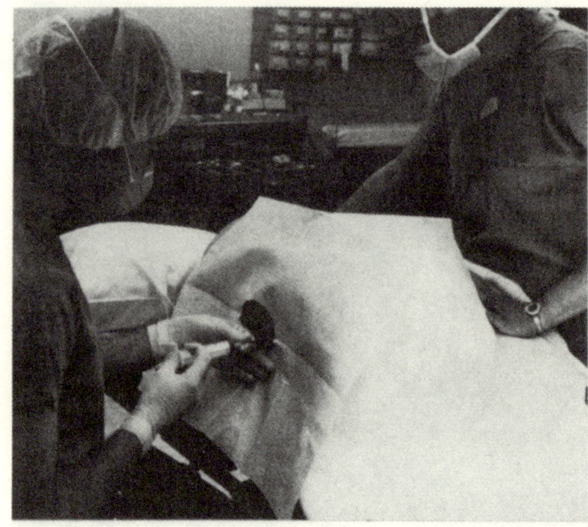

Barbara is draped, and her epidural is given.

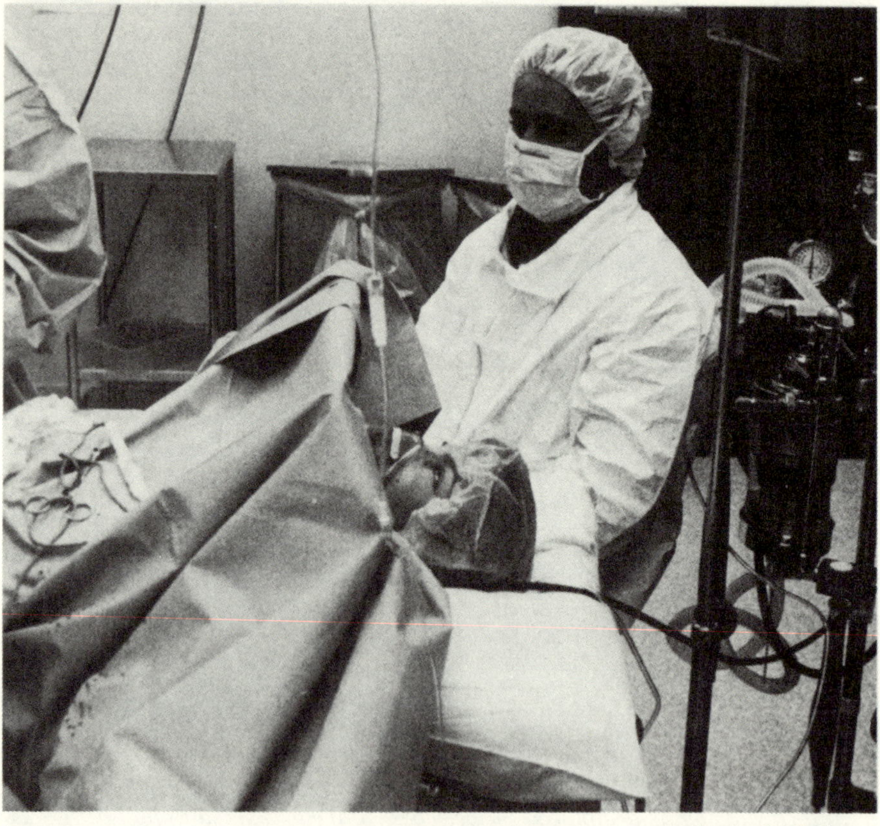

The doctors prepare Barbara's abdomen for surgery. An anesthetic shield is set up to separate off the sterile surgical area. Oxygen is administered. Jack is seated at Barbara's head.

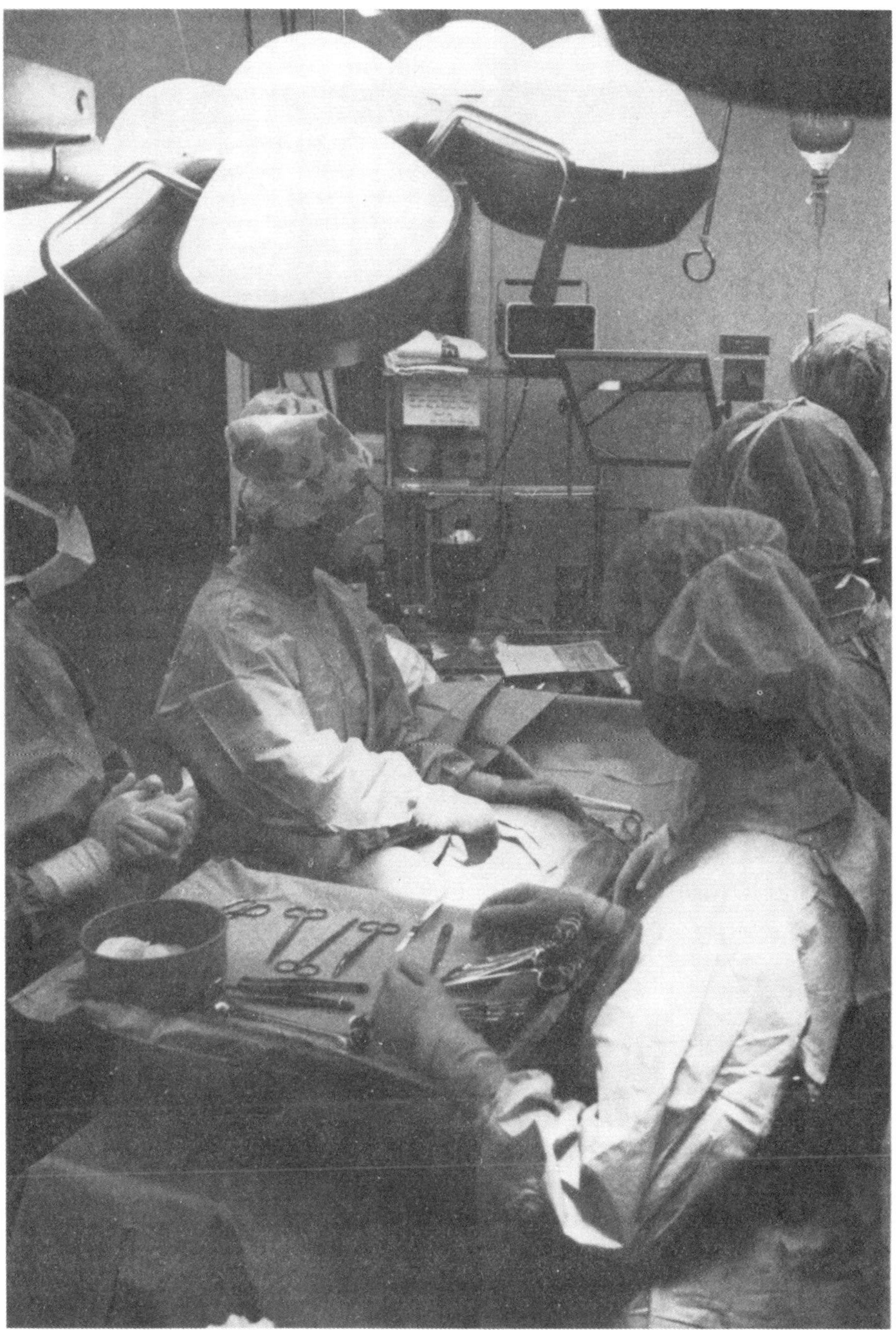

It will only take about five minutes until the baby is born. Barbara is aware of some tugging and pulling sensations. The doctor cuts several layers of tissue before reaching the uterus.

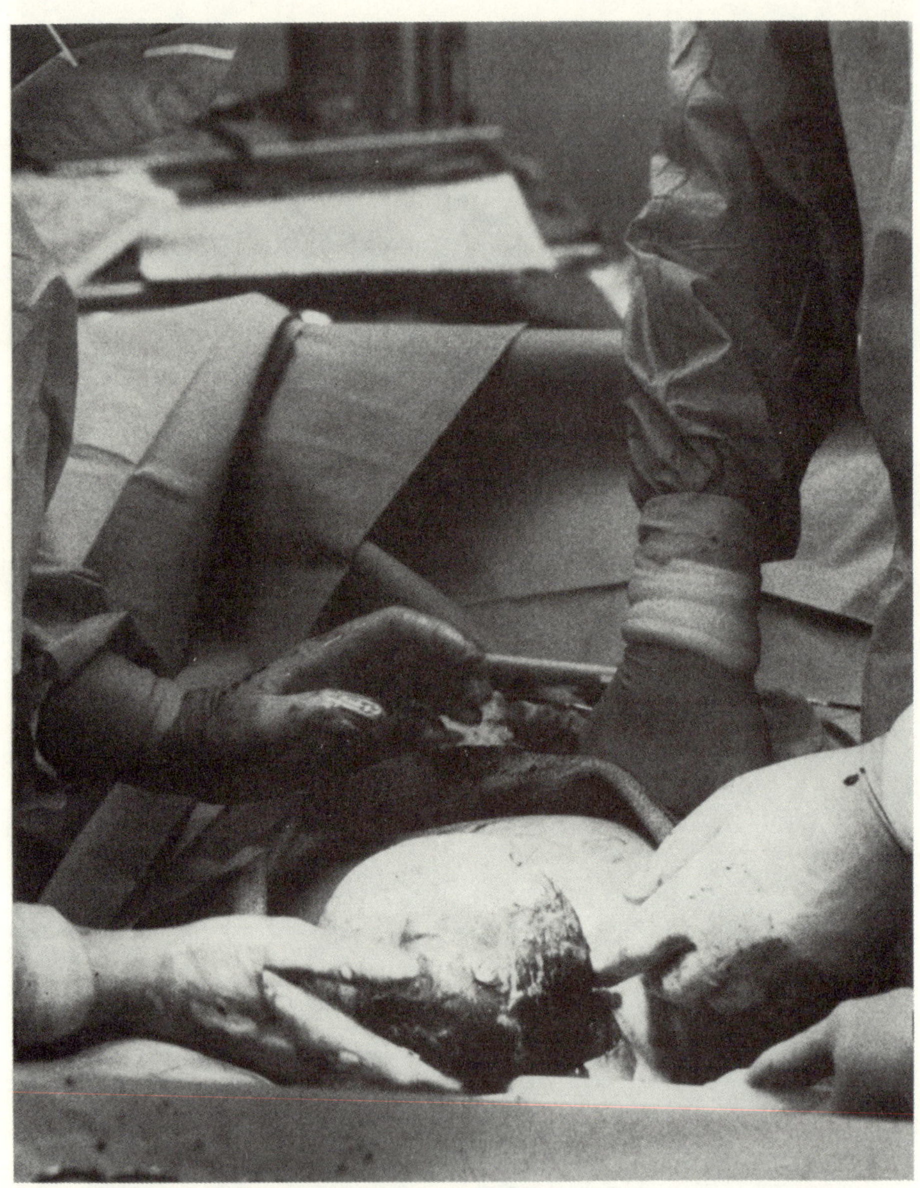

When the doctor cuts the uterus, the bag of waters will be broken and the amniotic fluid will come gushing out. If it does not break, the doctor will make a small opening in the bag and suction the fluid out with a catheter. Then he will pull out the baby's head.

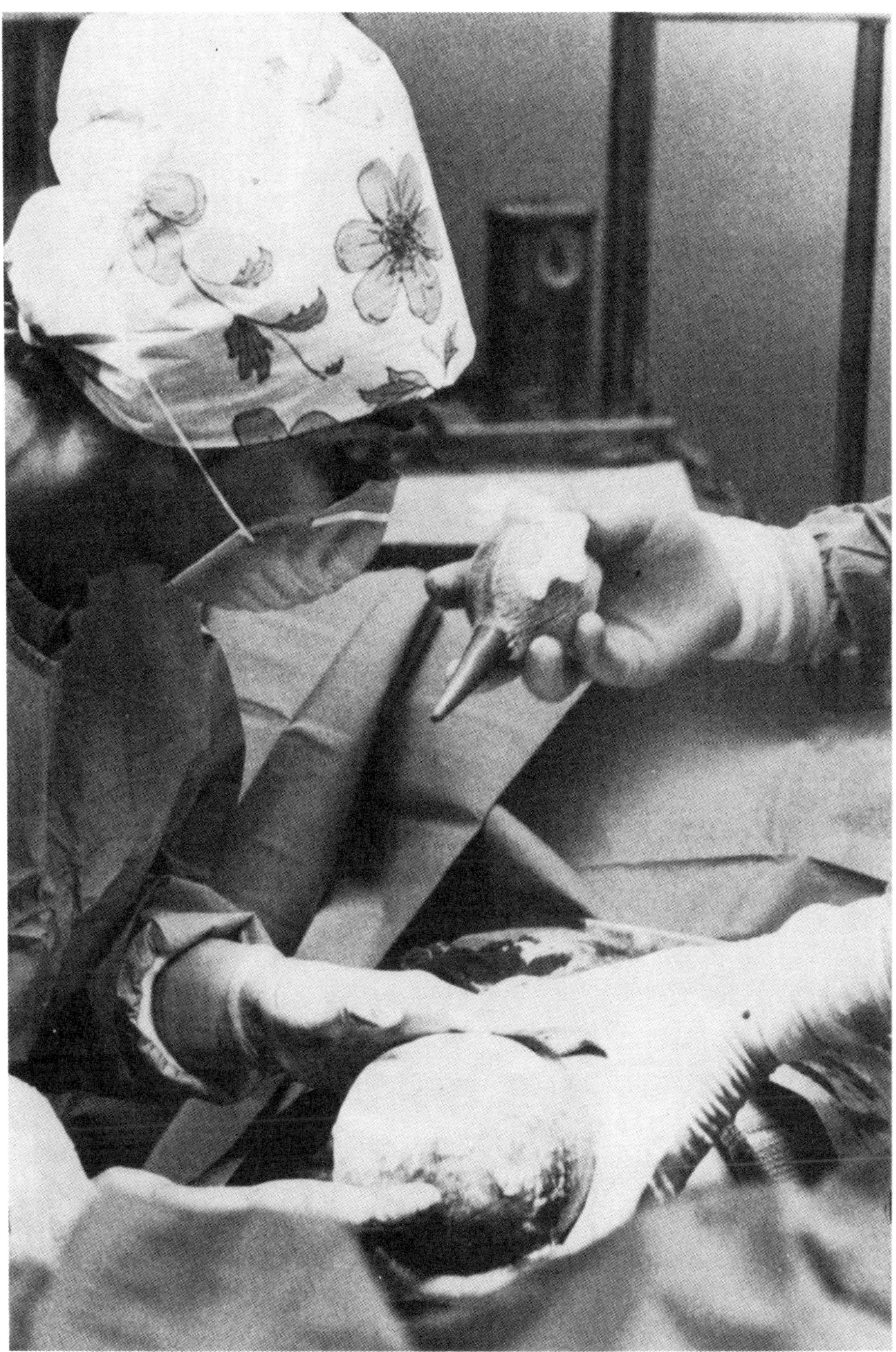

The doctor says, "Stand up, Jack, your baby is being born." Barbara can feel the tugging.

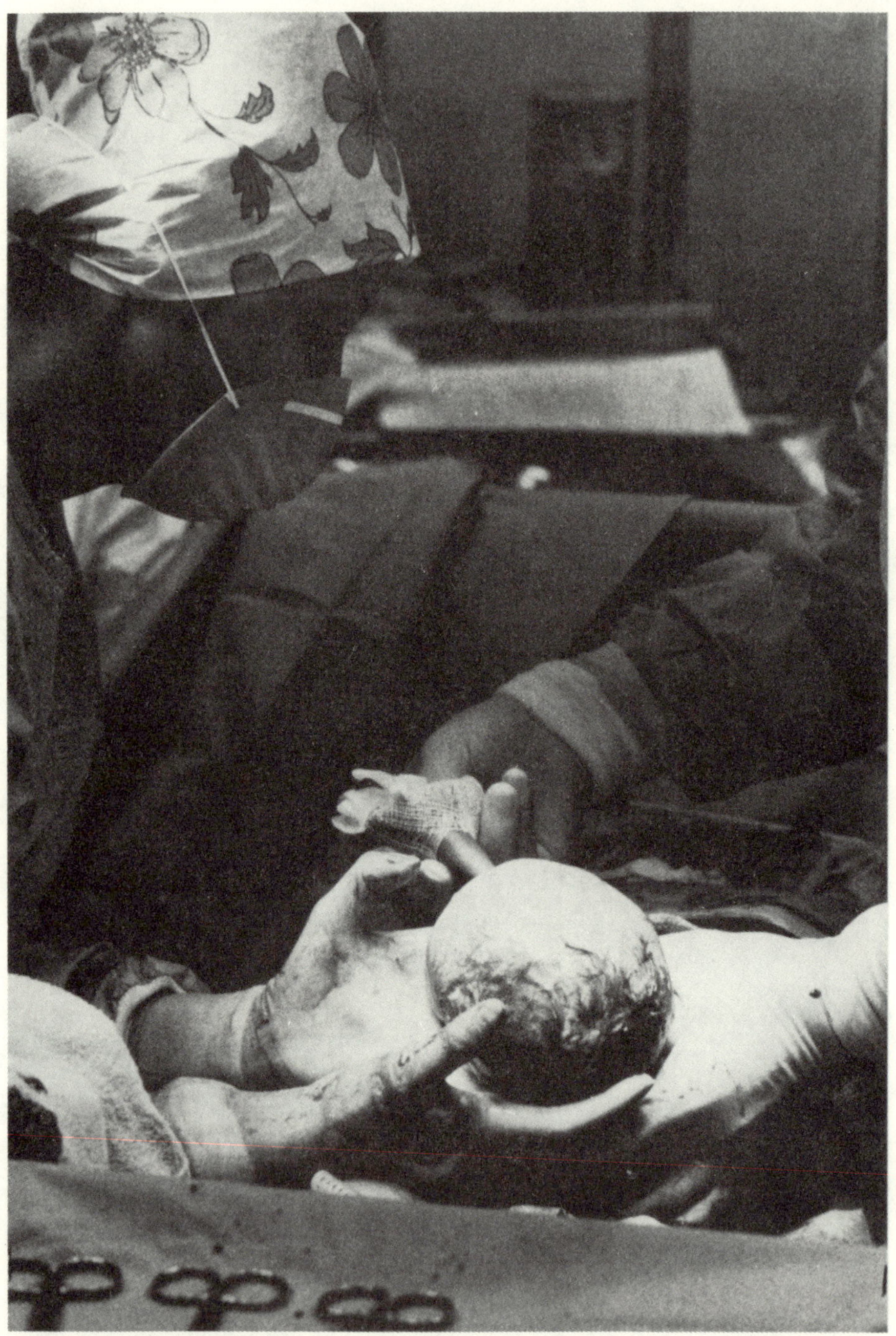

As soon as the head is out, the doctor suctions the baby's mouth and nose to clear its airway passages.

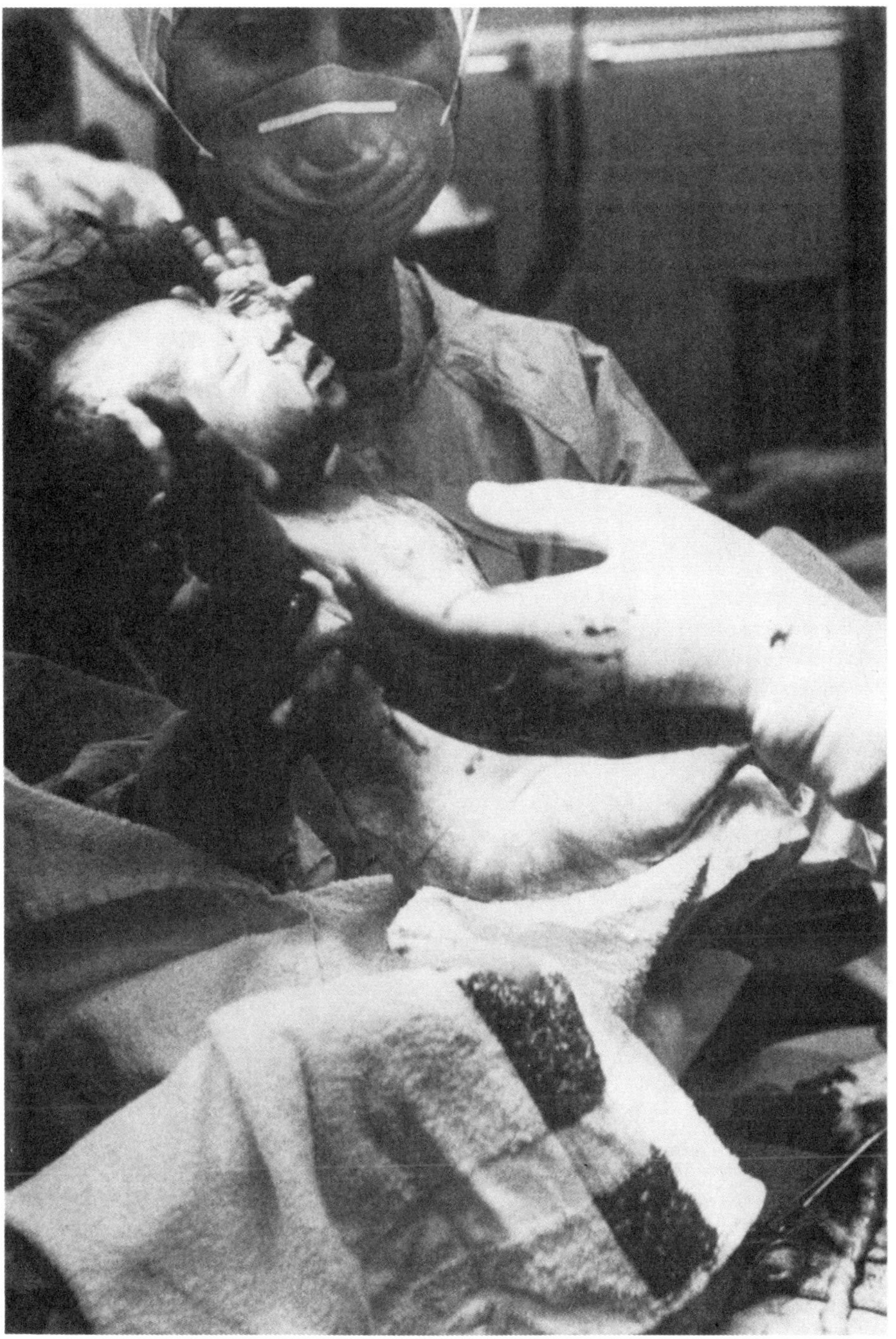

"It's a boy."

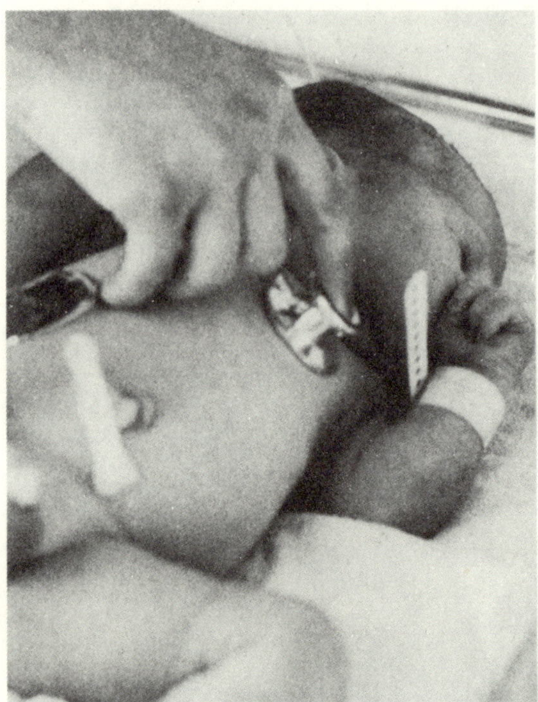

The doctor immediately cuts the cord and gives the baby to the pediatrician for a brief examination. Both parents can watch.

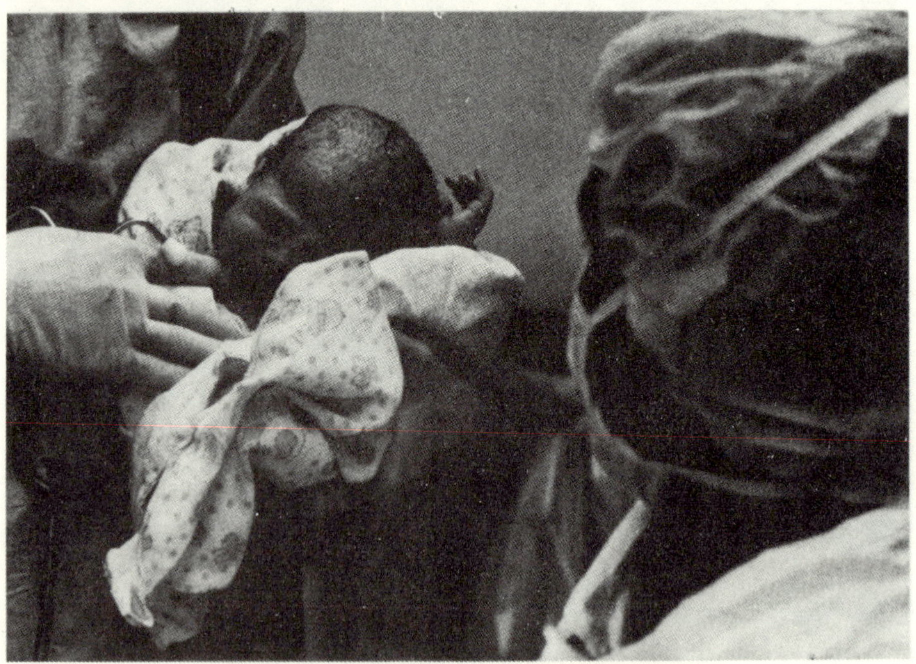

The pediatrician gives Aran to his parents.

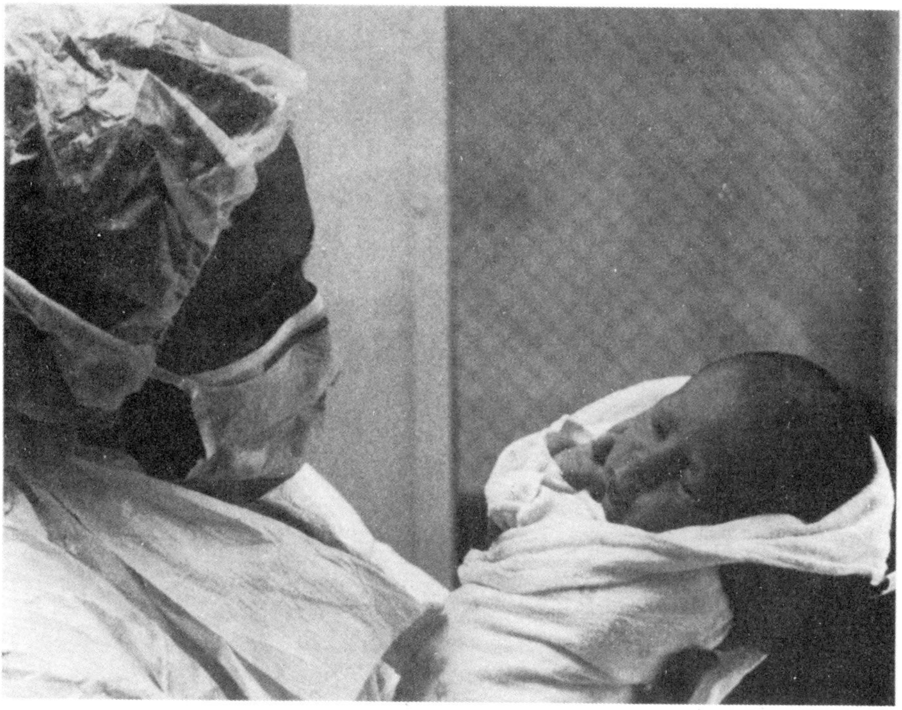

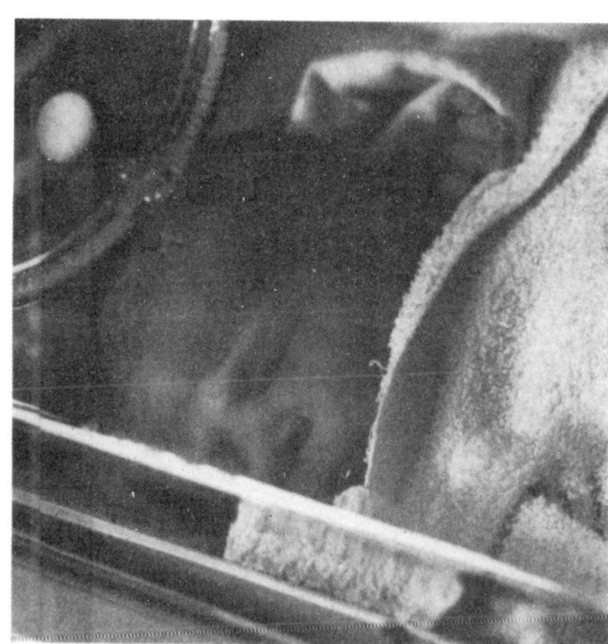

Seeing your newborn baby is a prime time for bonding.

Barbara can watch Aran while the doctors finish closing the incision.

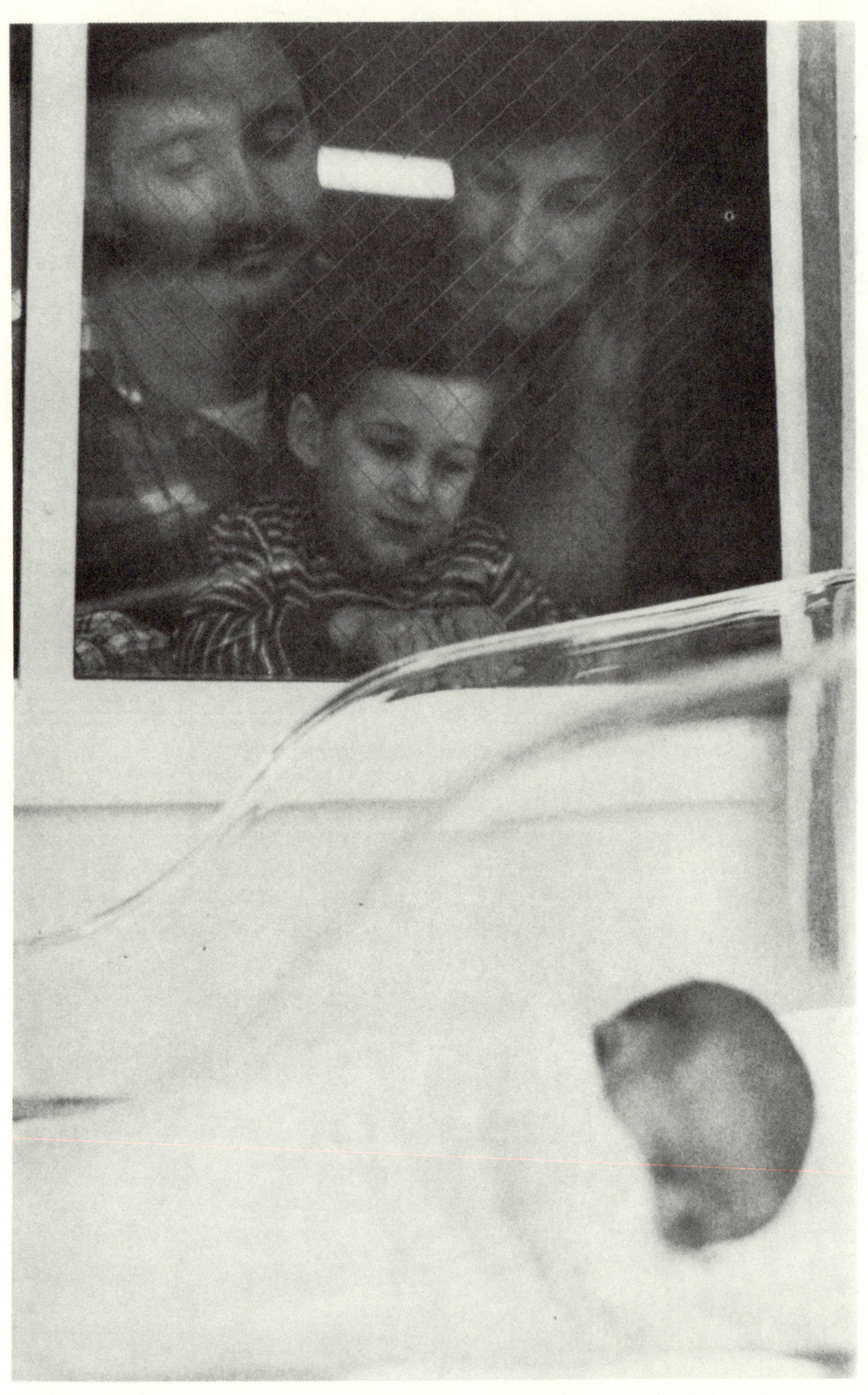

Barbara and Jack have shared a cesarean birth that has enriched their lives.

PART IV
After the Birth

CHAPTER TWELVE

Cesarean Postpartum Care

The days immediately following surgery will be days of physical and emotional upheaval. Given a little time, your body will adjust. However, there are things you can do to hasten your recovery and make your stay in the hospital more comfortable. The time you spend in the hospital can vary from about three days to two weeks, but the average stay for a cesarean mother is five to seven days. The amount of time you spend in the hospital will depend on your doctor's preference and your physical condition. Don't be in a hurry to leave the hospital.

REST—YOUR BEST MEDICINE

The most important thing you can do for yourself is to rest. The hospital routine and your new baby will keep you busy, so you will be wise to limit the number of visitors and phone calls you receive daily. You can ask the hospital operator to hold your calls for any period of time you wish. Your mate can suggest to family and friends that they not visit for the first two days. He should remind them to keep their visits short, because you tire easily. Your physical and emotional stability go hand in hand. Therefore, if you are rested you are less likely to suffer from postpartum depression or "baby blues." You will have more energy to cope with the stress and discomfort common to a new cesarean mother. A rested mother will be able to enjoy being with her baby and husband.

EXERCISE—MORE GOOD MEDICINE

Equally important to your speedy recovery is faithful exercise. You should continue the abdominal exercises you began in the recovery room. As mentioned earlier, this will aid tremendously in warding off the gas pains that plague abdominal surgery patients. It is hard to get in the frame of mind to do your exercises right after surgery, but the importance of doing so cannot be stressed too much.

Move around in bed as often as you can. Even if you have had spinal anesthesia and are required to lie flat in bed for several hours, you can and must move around. Moving facilitates circulation of blood to all parts of the body, including the wound, which in turn promotes healing of the incision. Moving also can prevent postsurgical complications such as pneumonia, urinary tract infections, and phlebitis (an inflammation of veins in the legs). Although these complications of cesarean surgery are rare, they do occur and can be avoided. Remember, moving decreases the likelihood of gas pains.

Initially, movement will be painful, but pain will decrease in the days to come. You should not lie flat on your back for long periods of time. The nurse will position you on your side, where you should remain for an hour or two. Ideally, you should change position from side to back to side at two-hour intervals. Your husband can help you change positions for the first few days when he is with you.

Moving your legs is particularly important in preventing phlebitis. You should pull your toes forward, press the backs of your knees into the bed, and exercise your ankles by making circles with your feet. These motions all require little physical exertion but are vitally important in keeping blood circulating in your legs. They should be done ten times an hour while you are awake for as long as you remain in the hospital. Stretch your arms, too.

Walking—The Big Challenge

During the first day, you will be walking with the aid of a nurse. *Do not attempt to walk alone until the nurse gives you permission to do so.* You will find that taking the first walk after surgery is a challenge. The nurse will show you how to inch over to the side of the bed —with the head of the bed raised as high as it will go—and how to swing your legs over the side of the bed. You should sit for a moment, take a deep breath, make sure you aren't dizzy, and then stand. The nurse will support you. Patients often feel they have no muscle support. Splint (support) your incision by placing your two hands over it, palms down, and press firmly. If your abdomen needs additional support, you can wear a light-weight girdle or abdominal binder. Ask the doctor or nurse about this.

Later you will be walking by yourself. You may still feel a pulling sensation at the incision. This sensation may make you want to stoop over and do the "cesarean shuffle." But your stitches won't split. *Stand tall.* You will look and feel better. *Now walk!* Up the halls, down the halls. Start a walking marathon with other cesarean mothers —a penny a mile, or whatever—but *walk.* This is the best thing you can do at this point in the recovery process to feel better fast.

POSTOPERATIVE DIET

You will be fed by IV (the intravenous needle in your hand or arm) immediately after surgery and until your intestines start to function again. With surgery, your intestines will stop normal functioning for a few days, but the IV will supply the nutriment your body requires. For the first twenty-four to thirty-six hours after delivery, many mothers receive nothing by mouth except ice chips. You will then graduate to a liquid diet. You can expect to be brought such delectables as broth, juices, and soda. The liquid diet is followed by a soft diet that is equally exciting, including gelatin, pudding, more broth, and tea. As soon as you have an adequate oral intake, the IV can be removed. The progression of your diet is up to your doctor. Some doctors order a full diet a day or two after surgery. Others wait until they hear bowel sounds when they listen to your abdomen with a stethescope. if your hear your stomach "growling" or gurgling, or if you pass gas, tell the nurse. This evidence that your intestines have resumed action will herald the coming of a more palatable meal!

NUTRITION AND HEALING

After surgery, your body will have a special need for protein, vitamin C, vitamin K, and the B vitamins. As previously discussed, protein is the building block of the body. Protein is essential for adequate healing of tissue. Be sure to continue to eat a minimum of four servings of protein daily.

Vitamin C is extremely helpful to the body when coping with stress. It also helps hold cells together and helps heal wounds. Vitamin C must be taken daily, because the body does not store it. Consult the chart in Chapter 3 for rich sources of vitamin C. Fresh fruits and vegetables are best; if not available fresh, they should be obtained frozen or canned.

Vitamin K is essential for the clotting of blood. Cabbage, cauliflower, spinach, other leafy vegetables, soybean oil, and other vegetable oils are sources of vitamin K. A vitamin K deficienty is rare if you are following a nutritional diet.

Whole-grain breads, cereals, and pasta are good sources of the B vitamins. Use only whole-grain products.

AVOIDING GAS

As mentioned before, an effect of adbominal surgery is the cessation of normal intestinal functioning. On about the second or third day, the intestines start working again, and this is when painful gas distension can occur. It will help to avoid carbonated beverages, drinking through a straw, apple juice, and drinking iced beverages. Ice chips, which will probably be offered the first few days, do not have the same effect as drinking an iced beverage and are quite refreshing, so don't turn them down! Avoid foods that normally cause you to form gas.

In addition to being careful about what you eat and drink, you may do the following to relieve gas pain: Lying on your *left* side, pull your knees up and massage your abdomen from right to left. Remember to move around in bed often and walk whenever you can. If this doesn't bring the desired relief, tell the nurse. She can give you a Harris flush, which is administered like an enema, or she can insert a flexible tube into the rectum to break up the gas and move it out through the tube.

DEALING WITH POSTOPERATIVE DISCOMFORT

Each woman's pain threshold is different. Some women have very little discomfort and seem to breeze right through even the first twenty-four hours; other women experience quite a bit of discomfort after a cesarean birth.

Afterpains are experienced following either vaginal or cesarean childbirth. They are felt when the uterus contracts, a normal phenomenon following birth. Such contractions are more intense when the baby sucks at the breast, because of oxytocin, a hormone that the mother secretes when the baby nurses.

Some women experience pain in their shoulders, caused by an accumulation of air and blood under the diaphragm. The discomfort occurs in the shoulder area rather than at the diaphragm because there are nerve connections between the two areas. This air and blood is gradually reabsorbed, and the pain will disappear.

Pain Medication—Take It

Of course, you cannot avoid having some pain, but taking pain medication will help control it. *Take your medicine—this is no time to be stoic.* When you begin to feel discomfort, call the nurse and request your medication. If you wait until the pain becomes intense, you will need more medication for relief. The doctor leaves orders for you to have specified medication, so don't hesitate to speak up. There are many different types of pain medication, so if you are experiencing any negative side effects, such as grogginess, ask to try something different.

Try to anticipate the times you will most need to be free of pain, and take your pain medication ahead of time, because the effects of the medication are not felt immediately. For instance, plan with your nurse to take your pain medication thirty minutes to an hour before walking for the first time. If you are nursing, another good time to take your medication is before the nurse brings you the baby to feed. It may be hard to nurse if you are tense with pain.

Pain medication will facilitate your recovery by helping you feel comfortable the first few days after surgery. If you are free from pain, you will do the things you need to do for your well-being. You will take those deep breaths, cough, move around in bed, and do your exercises. If you are in pain you may opt to just lie in bed perfectly still. If you are comfortable, you will sleep better and be rested and relaxed enough to enjoy and get to know your new baby. You and your husband can also better enjoy this special time together if you are not in pain.

LOCHIA (VAGINAL FLOW)

After delivery, *every* new mother must contend with lochia, or vaginal flow of blood. This is the wall of the uterus sloughing off, just as it does each month with menstrual cycles. It will be bright red for the first three or four days and then will gradually turn yellow white after two or three weeks. Lochia is an excellent criterion for early detection of internal problems. Notify your doctor if your flow suddenly increases, if you find any clots, or if the lochia develops a bad odor.

COUGHING—GRIN AND BEAR IT

You should cough every hour during your hospital stay. Coughing and deep breathing get air into the far corners of the lungs, thus preventing pneumonia, which is a possible complication of any surgery. After surgery, when the patient is feeling uncomfortable and not exerting herself, she tends to use only part of the lungs. The air sacs not being used can become closed with mucus. Coughing and deep breathing keep them open. If it hurts to cough, hold your incision with your hands, or hold a pillow firmly over your abdomen to support your incision.

SPEAK UP

As the nurses care for you, much will be happening that you will not understand. Don't be afraid to ask questions. The nurses and doctors are there to help you. However, they cannot read your mind, so if there is something troubling you or if there is something you want to know more about, *speak up*.

One more word of advice. Concentrate on yourself for the first forty-eight hours. You have had major surgery, and you need coddling. Don't feel as if you have to be Supermother and put unrealistic demands on yourself. If you are nursing, it is a good idea to do so as early as possible, but let the nurse help you. When your husband is with you, he can position the baby for you, and later he can hold and burp the baby.

EMOTIONS

For too long, doctors, hospital staff, and the public in general have substantially ignored the emotional needs of the cesarean mother. Fortunately, in the last few years we have experienced a new awareness of the human aspects of the birthing process. Your emotional welfare also needs nurturing. This is particularly true if you have had an emergency cesarean childbirth instead of the natural one you had planned. You may be feeling many negative emotions, such as disappointment, failure, bewilderment, and guilt. It will help if you can talk about these feelings. Verbalize how you feel to your husband, your doctor, or anyone else who will listen. Other cesarean mothers will only be too eager to talk with you. This will bring your feelings out into the open, where you can examine them and reconcile yourself to what has happened. You may want to contact a local cesarean support group. It is a rewarding experience to meet and exchange experiences and feelings with other couples who have gone through a similar experience. Keep in mind that if you did not enjoy a father-attended cesarean birth this time, you can plan for one for your next baby and have a totally different experience.

Postpartum Depression

Postpartum depression, more commonly referred to as "baby blues," affects over a hundred thousand women a year. It usually lasts one to seven days. Women suffering from this depression complain of feeling low, restless, tired, irrritable, dissatisfied, tearful, and anxious. It is a common, and not unexpected, phenomenon.

Doctors believe that postpartum depression may be caused by a hormone imbalance. During pregnancy there is a gradual change in the hormone balance, but during the postpartum period the hormone changes take place more rapidly and can have a direct bearing on your emotional state.

A factor of a nonbiological nature that may influence postpartum depression is lack of emotional support. It is important to a woman at this time to have the love and understanding of the father and/or other family members. If she doesn't have this, then the support of a good friend will help. Unfortunately, in some cases there is no one who will provide support. If you are in such a situation, consider contacting a local cesarean support group or your clergyman.

Your own personality is also a factor influencing the degree of postpartum depression you might experience. A person who is generally easy going will perhaps react differently than a person who is normally high-strung.

Other factors contributing to postpartum depression can include the amount of stress in your life, role expectations, nutritional deficiency, exhaustion from the cesarean, and any negative feelings you may have about your cesarean delivery. The main thing to remember is that it is largely a hormone imbalance, and it will correct itself in about a week.

However, some steps you might take to help yourself while you wait for this condition to pass, or to minimize the depression would include:

1. Don't repress your feelings. If you have a lot of negative feelings, let them out, don't dwell on them. Try positive thinking and concentrate on subjects that normally are pleasant to you.

2. Don't set unreasonably high goals for yourself. Remember that you are convalescing from major surgery as well as undergoing

hormonal changes that are affecting your emotions as well as your body. Pamper yourself without guilt.

3. Avoid stressful situations. If your mother-in-law makes you nervous, perhaps your husband can tactfully run interference.

4. Get plenty of rest and sleep. If you are breastfeeding, this is often hard to do because the baby is brought to you every couple of hours around the clock. You would be wise to restrict visitors, forget addressing those birth announcements for now, and eliminate anything else that you can from your routine.

When you are no longer receiving intravenous feedings, you should eat the hospital food that is served to you even if it sometimes does not appeal to you. You might ask the nurse to bring you something else. Please remember that you do need to eat well.

If you feel like crying, cry. And don't apologize just because you can't tell what you're crying about. Baby blues are no fun, but fortunately, given a little time, they pass away and leave you feeling like your old self again.

If, after a month, you are still feeling depressed or you experience the following symptoms of severe depression, you should seek professional help: difficulty sleeping night after night; helpless feelings, such as feeling you can't face the day; avoiding contact with everyone including your own family; inability to make simple decisions or perform simple tasks such as car-pooling or going to the market; loss of interest in food and sex; and constant unhappiness. If some of these symptoms persist, you are not suffering from ordinary "baby blues," and you must see a doctor or mental health professional.

CHAPTER THIRTEEN

Breastfeeding and Bottlefeeding

Having myself experienced a wide variety of attitudes toward breast-feeding during the ten-year span over which I had my three children, I feel I can relate to women who want to breastfeed, who feel indifferent, or who do not want to breastfeed.

When I was twenty-three and pregnant for the first time, I was taken completely by surprise when my doctor asked me, "Are you going to breastfeed or bottle-feed your baby?" I honestly hadn't considered the question. I suppose if I had been living in a time when most women breastfed their babies as a natural way of life, I probably would have just taken it for granted that I would, too. The doctor would have probably made the same assumption. However, in the 1940s and 1950s, it became unfashionable to nurse babies. Only about one-third or less women nurse their offspring in this country. I replied to the doctor, "I don't know. What do you think I should do?" The doctor seemed indifferent. "It's really up to you. If you do plan to breastfeed, I will need to put it on your chart." I didn't feel it mattered much to him.

I went home. I asked my husband after dinner, "Do you think I should breastfeed the baby?" The question apparently also caught him by surprise. "Gee, honey, that's up to you. Won't breastfeeding tie you down even more?" He didn't seem very enthusiastic.

I didn't have any close friends with babies. My mother lived in another city, and she had not breastfed me so I didn't think it would be very helpful to call her. I felt vaguely threatened by the idea of breastfeeding. I may have felt my husband wouldn't think I was sexy any more. I also thought it might be painful and messy. I decided not to nurse. As it turned out, I had a surprise cesarean and I felt sure I had made the right decision. After all, cesarean mothers can't nurse anyway! At least, that's what everyone said.

The second time I became pregnant, I was more open to the idea of breastfeeding. I asked the doctor about it, and he discouraged me because I was going to have a repeat cesarean. He thought the disadvantages outweighed the advantages. I really didn't know what the advantages were, having never read anything about breastfeeding. Also, I was not fortunate enough to know anyone who was in favor of breastfeeding to instruct and encourage me on the subject. Again, I decided not to breastfeed.

The third time I became pregnant, breastfeeding was finally becoming popular. Much was being written on the subject to educate young mothers to the benefits and advantages of nursing. These books and magazine articles did much to dispel fears and encourage women to breastfeed. I was lucky to have friends who were enthusiastic about breastfeeding. One breastfeeding promoter gave me the wonderful book distributed by *La Leche League, The Womanly Art of Breastfeeding.*[1] Another friend gave me Karen Pryor's book, *Nursing Your Baby,* which is also excellent.[2] I decided I wanted to try it. I told my doctor I intended to nurse this baby and asked him to put that fact on my chart so there would be no mistake at the hospital. Nursing my last baby was so easy, natural, healthy, and enjoyable that I sincerely wish I had nursed all my children. It's amazing, when you think about it, that we could have come to the point in our culture at which a woman must read books, find encouragement from friends, and make special arrangements at the hospital to perform such a simple, God-given bodily function as nursing one's own newborn.

CAN CESAREAN MOTHERS BREASTFEED?

The answer is yes! Breastfeeding is natural for any woman. Surgery does not affect the flow of mother's milk. Hormonal changes associated with pregnancy are responsible for producing milk. The mode of delivery has nothing to do with the production of the milk.

The idea that cesarean mothers can't breastfeed comes from a time when cesarean childbirth was treated strictly as surgery, not childbirth. Cesarean mothers were kept in hospital beds for weeks, and they convalesced slowly. Doctors at that time felt that "sectioned" mothers couldn't nurse. In recent years, the trend has been for early ambulation (walking), which facilitates early recovery and resumption of strength and bodily functions. Occasionally we hear of a doctor that still has the notion a cesaren mother shouldn't nurse. This idea may be a carryover from the past.

There are some reasons why a cesarean mother might develop a problem that would prevent her from nursing; however, these occurrences are rare. We will discuss these exceptions later in this chapter.

Breastfeeding has some special advantages for cesarean mothers. Psychologically, breastfeeding after a cesarean delivery is very consoling. If you feel disappointed that you could not deliver vaginally, it is reassuring to know that you can feed the baby naturally. For most women, breastfeeding is pleasurable. Breastfeeding offers the cesarean mother an excellent opportunity to establish a bond of trust and affection between herself and the infant. She can feel glad, knowing she is giving the baby the best milk possible. Also, nursing stimulates the uterus to contract and resume its normal size, an important factor in recovering from surgery.

BENEFITS FOR THE BABY

The nutrient content of breast milk is uniquely suited for your baby. It is easily digested and easier for the baby's immature liver and kidneys to handle. The concentration and types of protein in the mother's milk are ideal for infant growth and are less likely to cause allergic reactions than other kinds of milk. Immunities are passed from mother to baby through mother's milk.

Human milk is high in cholesterol. This may seem to be unhealthy, because cholesterol is sometimes considered a "villain" in heart disease. Actually, cholesterol plays an important role in the proper development of the newborn's nervous system. It is thought that when the baby is exposed to high levels of cholesterol during infancy he develops methods to control cholesterol in a healthy way. Thus, exposure to high levels of cholesterol from breast milk may be important in preventing problems with cholesterol in adulthood.[3]

There are other advantages to nursing. Breast milk is clean and not easily contaminated. Breastfeeding provides protection against obesity. The baby knows when its stomach is full. Bottle-fed babies are encouraged to drain the last drop from the bottle. They are sometimes given an extra bottle they do not even want, just to satisfy their sucking instincts. Breastfed babies have a soft, odorless, almost liquid stool, which is easy to pass. A bottle-fed baby is more prone to straining and constipation.

Breastfeeding requires no buying, mixing, or preparation. You cannot make mother's milk too weak or too strong by diluting incorrectly. And breast milk is always the right temperature. You never have to heat it or be concerned that it is too hot or not warm enough. Breast milk is always fresh and convenient. Finally, breastfeeding is economical.

BENEFITS FOR THE MOTHER

Breastfeeding helps get you back into shape after the birth, because it causes the uterus to contract, via the secretion of oxytocin. Breastfeeding can also prevent or stop hemorrhaging. In areas of the world where prolonged breastfeeding is practiced, the incidence of breast cancer is low. Indeed, studies show that there is a lower likelihood of breast cancer in women who breastfeed.

Studies have also shown that complete breastfeeding for the first four to six months has an effect on natural spacing of pregnancies because it postpones the resumption of ovulation and the menstrual cycle for seven to fifteen months. This does not mean you cannot become pregnant while you are nursing, but it is extremely rare to become pregnant before the first menstrual period if the mother is nursing fully. However, if you wish to avoid or postpone another pregnancy, be sure to discuss an appropriate method of contraception with your doctor.

COMMON CONCERNS

Many women worry that nursing will ruin the shape of their breasts. This is not true; in fact, nursing may well improve the shape of your breasts. If you wear a good supportive bra, you should have no problem with "sagging breasts." Concern is often expressed by new mothers that their breasts are not the right size or shape to nurse a baby. You need not worry about this—the size of the breast has nothing to do with your ability to make or store milk. Flat or inverted nipples can be difficult until you and the baby work out a solution. You may need to use a nipple shield in the beginning until the baby learns to "take hold."

Also, don't worry about whether your milk will be rich enough. Mother's milk is almost always best suited for the baby. Of course, you should make an effort to eat nutritious food, but even if your diet is not very good your milk will, in most instances, be better than baby formula. Don't be deceived by the appearance of the milk. It may resemble nonfat milk—thin and bluish—but that's the way it is supposed to look.

You may be concerned about producing enough milk. You will

produce ample milk if you keep the baby at your breast long enough at each nursing session. The more the baby nurses, the more milk your breast produces. If your supply of milk does not satisfy the baby's hunger, you may have to feed him more often until your breast builds up its store of milk.

New nursing mothers also become concerned about what will happen if they become ill. You don't have to stop nursing if you come down with the common cold or flu. The baby will no doubt have been exposed before you realized you were getting sick. As we mentioned before, your breast milk has built-in immunities to infection and is the best thing for the baby under these circumstances. The same principle applies if the baby gets sick. Breast milk is the best thing for him.

You may wonder if you could be too nervous to nurse. Extreme nervousness can affect the "letdown" reflex (discussed later) so that the milk is not released. The milk supply is there, however, and the milk will come down as soon as you relax. Keep the baby at your breast and be a little patient. Sometimes drinking a beer while nursing can help your to relax.

Because the cesarean mother is at the hospital longer than mothers who have had vaginal deliveries, she gets more help from the experts before going home. If you are having a struggle with anything, such as nerves, pain, letdown reflex, inverted nipples, and so on, the nursing staff can give you the assistance and reassurance you need. Just be sure to voice any worries or problems.

DIFFICULTY WITH BREASTFEEDING

Some women cannot nurse their babies. The basic cause for almost every breastfeeding failure is failure of the letdown reflex. The milk is there, but the mother cannot give it to the baby until the functioning of a reflex within the breast called the "letdown reflex." The letdown reflex occurs when the milk-secreting lobes of the breast, which wrap around the alveoli and duct wall, contract. The reflex pushes the milk down into the main breast cavities right under the nipple. When this happens, the baby effortlessly removes the milk by suction. The milk almost pours into the baby's mouth. A baby doesn't need strong suction to remove the milk; he only needs to fit the nipple into his mouth so that he compresses the areola (the dark area around the nipple) and the milk will flow out.

The letdown reflex is a physical response to a physical stimulus. Why, then, is failure of the letdown reflex the basic cause of almost every breastfeeding failure? The answer is that this reflex is greatly affected by the mother's emotions. Any disturbance, particularly in the early days of lactation, can inhibit the letdown reflex. Such stresses as embarrassment, irritation, or anxiety actually prevent the pituitary gland from secreting oxytocin, a hormone that stimulates the letdown reflex. Thus, a woman who dislikes breastfeeding, or is very much afraid she will fail, may give less milk than the mother who is interested and hopeful of success. A strong disturbance, such as real anger or fear, may send adrenalin through the system, causing the small blood vessels to contract so that oxytocin, even if released, does not reach the basket cells that let the milk down.[4]

How do you handle a faulty letdown reflex? First, while you are in the hospital don't begin to worry if you do not experience a letdown reflex as soon as you think you should. The nurses will be weighing your baby daily, and they will not let the baby lose too much weight or get hungry. The baby has fluid reserve to fall back on. This fluid reserve is why babies often look like "chubby cherubs" when they are born. You can encourage letdown by giving your baby the breast as early and as regularly as you can. The next thing to do is just relax and enjoy the baby, knowing that nature will take its course. If you feel that any situation at the hospital is causing stress, such as too much company, or the nurses rushing your time with the baby, or whatever, tell the nurses and ask them to change those conditions. Medications also can help. You may need pain medication or a mild tranquilizer to help you relax. If you know when you will be given the baby for the feeding, you can request the medication about twenty minutes before, so that the medication can take effect by baby's dinnertime.

When a mother's circumstances or anxiety make her particularly slow to let down her milk, some doctors prescribe 0.5 to 1.0 cc of oxytocin to be administered in a nasal spray just before each feeding. The oxytocin is quickly absorbed through the nasal membranes, and the milk lets down unfailingly. The emotional interference is bypassed, and the mother's self-produced letdown becomes conditioned. (One mother reported that by the second week her milk began to let down as soon as she picked up the nasal spray bottle.[5]

PREPARING YOUR NIPPLES BEFORE THE BABY ARRIVES

You can't really know until you have begun to nurse your baby if your are going to experience sore nipples. Many women never do anything to prepare or "toughen up" their nipples beforehand and never experience a moment's discomfort from sore nipples. Other women, particularly those with fair skin, do have difficulties with tenderness and soreness. Because you can't know ahead which category you will fall into, you would be wise to try to prevent this condition by proper care during pregnancy.

You don't need to do anything with the nipples for at least the first six months of your pregnancy. In the last three months, go easy on the soap when you are taking your bath and rinse off the soap well. In fact, you might stop using any soap at all. Your skin naturally secretes oils that help make the nipples strong and pliable. Scrubbing removes this protective oil, which is also antibacterial, making your breast more subject to dryness. Dryness can cause cracked nipples. To lubricate your breasts, you can use baby oil or cold cream.

HAND EXPRESSING MILK

It is sometimes recommended that you hand-express (press out) a few drops of colostrum from each breast every day during the last six weeks of pregnancy, and you may want to do this, with your doctor's approval. Colostrum is the fluid secreted before the milk comes in. Doctors agree that colostrum is very important for the newborn baby and is one good reason why you should nurse your baby as soon after delivery as possible. Expressing the colostrum daily for a few weeks before the baby is born opens the milk ducts, reducing the engorgement that sometimes occurs when the milk first comes in and that some mothers find quite uncomfortable.

Hand expression is quite simple. The method is the same for expressing colostrum during pregnancy or for expressing milk later on. First wash your hands. Then cup the breast in your hand, placing your thumb above and forefinger below the breast at the edge of the dark area (areola), and simply squeeze thumb and finger together gently. Don't slide the finger and thumb out toward the nipple. Don't worry if nothing comes out the first few times you try it. You'll get the knack soon. Rotate your hand slightly back and forth several times in order to reach all the milk ducts, which radiate out from the nipple.[6]

Nipples are tender because they are always protected from the elements by clothing, usually the soft lining of a bra. If you rarely wear a bra, then you have the advantage of tougher nipples. (Pregnant women will want to wear a bra for support so that later they will not have "sagging breasts.")

A Connecticut clinic found a simple solution for desensitizing the nipples while wearing a supportive bra. Trim a circle of material from the tips of the cups of your bras so that the nipple is exposed. Normal chafing against clothing will quickly toughen the nipple. (Stitch around the opening to prevent the cloth from unraveling.)[7]

Some women have flat or inverted nipples. One exercise often recommended is to pull out the nipple firmly a couple of times daily. The most convenient time is when you are dressing or undressing or taking a bath. You don't need to start this exercise until the last month of pregnancy. Hormones produced in pregnancy will also help the shape of the nipples to be more suitable for nursing.

Many women have flat nipples, but few women have truly inverted nipples. The best treatment for bringing out truly inverted nipples is the use of Woolwich breast shields, worn during pregnancy before the baby is born. Sometimes a mother may discover after the baby is born that she has an inverted nipple she never suspected, or (more often) that her nipples may be temporarily retracted because of engorgement. Worn between feedings, the Woolwich shields may be useful for this problem, too. If the problem is simply engorgement, wearing the shields for just the time between two feedings may do the trick. In more severe cases, it may be necessary to wear them for a day or two or even for two or three weeks. The mother should not save the milk that leaks into the shields to feed the baby, and she should wash the shields frequently with hot soapy water, rinse thoroughly, and dry carefully. She should try to leave the nipples exposed to the air for fifteen to thirty minutes several times each day.[8]

BREASTFEEDING IN THE HOSPITAL

Obviously because you have just had surgery you are in as much need of tender loving care as your newborn is. You may not feel like doing or be able to do everything for your baby at first. You will have your hands full just trying to care for yourself. You will be grateful for all the nursing care and medication you will receive. This trying period passes quickly, though, and you will find yourself able, and wanting, to do more and more for the baby.

One cesarean mother shared her hospital experience:

I was convinced my baby wasn't getting any milk the first day I tried to nurse. This made me very nervous and scared. I asked the nurse to give my baby a bottle. She explained to me that the baby was getting colostrum from me. "Colostrum," she said, "is the fluid in the milk glands before the milk comes in. It is good for the baby and all she needs for now." She explained that the true milk wouldn't come for days. She told me that they weighed Sarah every day, that Sarah was not losing weight and that everything was fine. I felt very relieved and decided to stick to breastfeeding. Sure enough, about two days later I felt the milk come in. I knew it was there. I could feel it. I was literally bursting with milk. It was exciting, and I felt very womanly and happy.

But, alas, I had all this milk, but when I tried to nurse, the baby could not get a grip on my nipple. She was making noisy, smacking sounds and fussing. She looked like she was working so hard and getting so frustrated. I tried and tried to help her, but I couldn't. Again, I was afraid I would have to give it up, I truly felt disappointed. I had felt so thrilled when my milk came in!

The nurse finally came and I asked her why we were having such a problem. "You have flat nipples," she told me. "Your breasts are full and hard with milk, and she cannot get hold." She tried to help me, but she could not succeed either. By now I was batting back the tears in my eyes. She left to get help. She soon returned with an apparatus that looked similar to a rubber nipple that goes on a baby bottle. She snapped it over my own flat nipple, and the baby took hold. I yelped "ouch" as the first surge of milk left my very full breast for Sarah's mouth. I felt the sensation of pain and sweet success all at the same time.

For the next two or three days, I nursed using this method. I wasn't hurting much any more, but I didn't like not having skin-to-skin contact with my baby. I resented having to use the rubber nipple. Realizing that I would soon be leaving the hospital and be more or less on my own, I decided to give my flat nipple one more try. When Sarah was brought to me I put the artificial nipple on just long enough to appease Sarah's appetite so she wouldn't panic if she had to work again for the milk. I also reasoned if my breast wasn't so full it would be more pliable. After Sarah nursed four or five minutes and we were both relaxed, I removed my hated rubber nipple and tried without it. Neither one of us knew exactly what to do, but we both had the same goal in mind. After some experimenting and struggling she got hold of me, locked on, and began to nurse. It felt so right. So good. Babies learn fast, even in a few days. She never had a problem getting hold of me after that even when I started out with a full breast. I realized that where there are will, love, patience, and confidence, there is a way![9]

This cesarean mother took advantage of her time in the hospital. She used this undisturbed time to work out a comfortable working relationship with her baby before she returned to the family routine at home. You, too, will experience the added advantage of having a knowledgeable and concerned medical staff to give you the help, and sometimes just the confidence, you need to assume total care of your newborn.

Cesarean mothers tell us all the time that nursing the baby is physically and emotionally a relaxing experience for a convalescing mother. The sooner you begin nursing after delivery, the better. If you are eager to begin nursing, be sure so tell your doctor how you feel so the nurses can arrange to get the baby to you as soon as possible.

BREASTFEEDING POSITIONS

Cesarean mothers often prefer to nurse lying down, which is easy and comfortable. When the nurse brings you the baby, tell her to lower the bed until it is almost flat and to leave the side rails up. Experiment with your pillows to discover what position gives you the most comfort and support. With the baby on his side and you on your side, have him placed with his mouth at your nipple, allowing your breast to touch his cheek. This will be a tender moment. You both may take right off, or it may be awkward and take some time to work it out. Either way, the final reward will be satisfying.

To burp the baby, roll him over onto your chest and rub his back. You don't need to pat him on the back to get the air bubble. Rubbing works better and is soothing to him. When changing position to the other side, hold him securely on your chest and roll over together.

Even if you have prepared your nipples for soreness, you are likely to feel a surge of momentary pain as the baby grabs the nipple and starts to suck. This pain eases away as the milk lets down.

Soreness generally starts around the twentieth feeding, gets worse for twenty-four to forty-eight hours, and then rapidly disappears. Sometimes the nipple looks a little red and chafed. It may crack or even bleed. The nipple will heal itself in spite of sucking provided that no harmful substances such as soap, alcohol, of petroleum jelly are applied. Keep the nipple dry and exposed to air between feedings. You can have someone bring you a couple of little sieves from dime-store tea strainers. You can put these in your bra. They will allow the air to circulate and keep you dry.

If your nipples are sore, keep on nursing. Start all feedings on the least sore side. Once the milk has let down, you can switch sides. If both sides are sore, express the nipple manually until the milk lets down. Remember to take your pain medication. Between feedings, soothe the nipples with hydrous lanolin.

Some maternity nurses suggest preventing sore, cracked nipples by timing your feedings for the first few days. The first day, nurse for one to five minutes by a clock, on each breast for each feeding. Then add one to two minutes each day.

Nursing is best accomplished on a reasonable demand schedule. An extremely helpful technique to ensure adequate milk supply is to nurse your newborn baby at least every 3 to 4 hours but not more often than every $1^{1}/2$ hours during the day. You may have to awaken the baby during the day to nurse if he sleeps longer than three to four hours. If the baby wishes to go longer between feedings at night, by all means do not discourage that! If you let your baby sleep for long periods during the day, you will probably find yourself up most of the night with a baby who has day and night mixed up.

To ensure ample milk supply for your baby, both breasts should be emptied at each feeding. This occurs when you follow the time guidelines just mentioned. However, if you allow your baby to "snack" whenever he cries by putting him to the breast, as many women do, you may find that you are nursing literally all day long—and feel really tied down by the nursing. More importantly, from the standpoint of adequate milk production, if the baby nurses too frequently he will just "top off" each time and never appreciably drain the breast. This discourages milk production. If the baby nurses too frequently, he will soon wake again, wanting a little more, and fall back to sleep again.

Babies often fall asleep while nursing because it is so warm next to Mom's skin and the warm milk satiates them. Be sure to wake your baby up between nursing at each breast by changing his diapers, stroking his back, or exercising his legs. When he is sufficiently awake, offer him the other breast. (Alternate which breast you offer first at each feeding.) In this way, the baby will be well fed, both of your breasts will be empty (which is a key to making plenty of milk), and your baby will be able to go longer between feedings. When the baby awakens, he will be very hungry and ready to empty the breasts again. This technique builds up a mother's milk supply.

In summary, a good rule is to nurse no sooner than $1^{1}/2$ hours after the last feeding and no longer than 3 hours after the last feeding during the day. Let the baby go as long as he wishes during the night.

Let the baby feed on "demand" within these guidelines. The entire nursing session should be limited to thirty minutes.

WORKING WITH THE NURSES

We have talked about many things you might want to do, or have done, while you are still at the hospital with your newborn. Some things we have suggested will be important to you, others will not. Just as each woman is different, so are hospital policies and nursing staffs.

In many hospitals, mealtime is rushed and the nurses don't have time to spend with each individual mother, but you will be surprised at how a smile, "please," "thank you," and a compliment can help you get around the busy routine. Be diplomatic. Compromises can be reached. The nurses will forgive you for upsetting their routine with your special requests. You, also, must remember that they are busy with other mothers and concerns and that they have rules that they must abide by. You can find out many hospital policies ahead of time.

In hospitals where everyone encourages breastfeeding, the nurses will be helpful to you at each feeding, and all your requests will probably be enthusiastically met. Whatever your situation, be calm. Your rewards will be a well-nourished baby and a feeling of personal satisfaction, richly deserved.

NUTRITION AND BREASTFEEDING

Breastfeeding your baby makes even greater demands on your body, in some respects, than does pregnancy. As the baby grows and becomes more active, the food supply from you must increase.

Your body goes through a total reorganization process as it adjusts from being pregnant to being not pregnant. During this time, your body is replenishing nutrient stores. It is also repairing and healing itself after the surgical delivery. Thus, if you are breastfeeding you must be conscientious about eating a nutritious diet.

Human milk consists of protein, sugar, and salts in which a variety of fatty compounds are suspended. In order to produce milk, your diet must contain an even higher number of calories (2,500 to 2,600 calories) while breastfeeding than it did during pregnancy. Also, you should drink 2 to 2 quarts of liquid daily. When you nurse, get a glass of juice, milk, or beer and put it beside you to drink. This is a good habit to ensure adequate fluid intake. If you are a vegetarian, you can

Daily Food Guide for Lactating Women

Food Group	Number of Servings
Protein foods	
Animal	2
Vegetable	2
Milk and milk products	5
Breads and cereals	4
Vitamin C fruits and vegetables	1
Dark Green Vegetables	1
Other fruit and vegetables	1

Source: California Department of Health, *Food Guides* (Sacramento: California Department of Health, 1977), p. 5.

nurse successfully by staying on the same well-balanced diet you practiced during your pregnancy.

If you are not conscientious about your diet, the consequences can be severe both for you and your baby. You may feel run down and may become prone to illness. Some women are extremely concerned about getting their slim figures back and thus restrict caloric intake after pregnancy. This can lower the quality of milk you produce and make your baby more vulnerable to health problems, particularly in the first few weeks of nursing. You will be wise to relax, eat well, and accept a gradual weight loss for the next six months to a year.

Drugs and Breastfeeding

If birth control pills are taken sooner than six weeks after the baby's birth, the amount of breast milk may be diminished. Talk to your doctor about other forms of birth control.

Other drugs, such as barbiturates, laxatives, and aspirin, can also be transmitted through breast milk. Again, check with your doctor before taking any drug.

Vitamins and Breastfeeding

While you are breast feeding, you need to supplement your diet with iron and folic acid. Also, a multivitamin pill is often prescribed by many doctors. Because breast milk does not contain an adequate amount of vitamin D, your pediatrician will probably prescribe vitamin D for you to give your baby. Depending on the fluoride content of the local water, the pediatrician may also suggest fluoride for the baby.

If you follow these recommendations, there is absolutely no reason why you will not provide an excellent and natural source of nutrition for your new baby's growth and development.

BOTTLE-FEEDING

If you decide to bottle-feed your baby, you have a variety of excellent modern formulas to choose from. Moreover, you will be able to convey the same love and warmth to your baby by bottle-feeding as by breastfeeding, although it will take a bit more conscious effort. One nice thing about bottle-feeding is that the father, grandparents, and other family members can share in this pleasurable activity. It can be a relief to you, as a cesarean mother recovering from surgery, to know that you are not the only one who can feed the baby. If you are bottle-feeding, you have more freedom to come and go because you are not tied to the feeding schedule. If you have someone to help you with the feedings, you can sleep through the night (or at least you may be able to sleep through some nights, depending on your arrangements). Even being able to sleep through the night every other day or so helps you get the rest you need.

Also, if you bottle-feed you escape any discomfort associated with breastfeeding, such as sore nipples. You also get back into your regular clothes faster. You don't have to worry about wearing clothes that provide easy access to the breast, or clothes that will be ruined if the milk should leak (pads, or Swedish nursing cups, will prevent milk from leaking onto your clothes).

For some women, it is important to see how much milk the baby is getting. Bottle-feeding affords this opportunity. The baby will go longer between feedings because the formula fills the baby for a longer period of time than does breast milk. In fact, formula babies occasionally demand too much milk and make themselves uncomfortable. For these reasons, we recommend a more regular schedule than for breast babies. You should wait at least $2^{1}/_{2}$ hours between feedings, and at night at least 4 hours.

Water should be offered between feedings to help with the schedule. If the baby has hard bowel movements, a tablespoon of dark Karo syrup in 4 ounces of water given two or three times a day is advisable. The baby will probably be hungrier on one day than the next, but you can usually rely on him to take the appropriate amount. The pediatrician will be checking and weighing the baby regularly, and he can advise you when to add solids to the baby's diet and which solids to include.

CHAPTER FOURTEEN

Home Again

Going home with the new baby you have waited nine months for is a happy time! It's a joy to take your newborn to the room that has been prepared for him with love and care. You have gone through the ritual a dozen times in your imagination, and now it's for real. It feels good to be in the privacy and warmth of your own home, surrounded by your family. It feels good to be free of hospital schedules and rules and to know you can hold your baby as long as you like without a nurse snatching him away. Because homecoming is a memorable event, you should savor every moment of it. You deserve to.

Part of the fun is sharing a new baby with his brother or sister. Usually children are excited and happy to have Mom home again and to have the chance to see and touch this mysterious little stranger. However, eager as they are to see you, they may harbor mixed emotions about having a new baby in the house. Some children have more positive feelings than negative ones. This helps make homecoming a high point in the birth experience. However, a child may feel threatened by the newcomer. He may feel uncertain about his own standing in the family unit. He may feel competitive and jealous. This is normal. If the child is handled with love and understanding, he will eventually change his negative behavior. In the meantime, he may ignore you or act hostile. So don't be surprised if he doesn't come running to your arms.

Don't worry so much ahead of time about an older child's reaction to the baby that the worrying spoils your homecoming. Some good advise is "Expect the best, and be prepared for the worst." Be sensitive to your child's reaction and play it by ear.

If you think your child will feel threatened by the baby when you arrive, it may be helpful to downplay the baby and give your other child your undivided attention. You might have a friend or relative take the older child out (to the park, for example). Meanwhile, you can come home with the baby and get him settled in bed. Then, when your other child comes in you can spend some time together, just the two or three (Daddy, too) of you. Try not to talk about the baby. You might be surprised how long it takes for your other child to bring up the subject of the new baby!

If the older child is at home when you arrive, have a family member carry the baby in while you make the reunion with your older child a special event. If there are relatives and friends present, ask them ahead of time to avoid excessive baby adoration. The newborn will never know he may have been slighted, but it will make a big difference to the older child.

The older child always seems to need something the minute Mom settles down to feed the baby. Try getting a snack, juice, and maybe a special toy for your child before you sit down to feed the baby. "Special toys" are old toys that you have put away out of sight for a few months. When they are pulled out again, they bring new delight.

You will notice that you are telling your older child, "*Wait just a minute, please!*" much more frequently than before the baby came. It is very helpful to tell the baby to wait sometimes, too. For example, if you are getting Susie a drink and the baby starts to cry, you might say, "Now, baby, I am getting your big sister a drink. You will have to wait a minute until I am finished." Kids love this.

Try to involve your older child in as much of the baby's care as he wishes—with supervision, of course. Babies are quite resilient, and with help an eighteen-month-old child can hold a newborn. Establish some firm rules: "If you want to hold the baby, get Mom or Dad first." The older child will typically lose interest after a few moments.

In his book *How to Parent*, Dr. Fitzhugh Dodson tells one mother's account of the reaction of a seventeen-month-old boy to his baby sister's birth:

When I first came home with Jenny, Mark stared at me first as though I were a complete stranger. He cried bitterly when his father carried Jenny from the car to the house. He was somewhat aloof for several hours. I was prepared to see some jealousy in Mark, but somehow I thought it would be subtle, or directed against me. Not so at all! The first chance he got he went right for the baby, with the most agonized expression, and tried to sock her. He looked grimly determined to smash this little bundle of trouble, and yet he was obviously terribly upset by his own impulse and sobbed, "No, no," even as he went for her. . . . The ice finally broke one day, perhaps a week after Jenny and I came home. I was diapering Jenny, and Mark was watching from his grandmother's arms. Jenny made some little noise. I imitated her and said to Mark, "Doesn't that baby make silly noises?" Suddenly Mark smiled broadly and said, "Silly!" It must have been a revelation to him that I was on his side. Here we were together, laughing at the baby. From then on, there was almost no more trouble.[1]

This story is a good illustration of a parent giving the child "permission" to express negative feelings toward the baby. Too often people think the thing to do is try to talk the older child out of his hostile feelings. We say things such as "Don't say you wish your brother would go away. You should love each other. Look, isn't he cute?" It is more helpful to feed the child's feelings back to him: "I see you do not like your brother right now. You would like him to go away. You feel Mommy loves him more than you." Such feedback tells the child you have heard, are not judging him, and are encouraging further communication.

It also helps for you to make some negative comments about the baby, such as "He sure does cry a lot, doesn't he!" Don't worry, your baby's feelings will not be hurt; but your older child will learn it's OK to express a negative feeling.

When children are not permitted to express their true feelings, they learn to internalize them. Show your child how to express negative feelings in a constructive way. If you have a preschool child, a baby doll is an excellent gift for either a son or a daughter. Preschool children, especially nonverbal ones, have rather primitive ways of expressing their feelings. The baby doll gives the child a healthy way to vent his feelings. If the child is feeling loving, he can imitate you and can pretend to bathe, dress, and diaper the baby. (This is also nice when the child is too young to participate in the newborn's real care.) If the child is feeling rebellious about the baby, he can act this out on the doll. Let him be as violent as he pleases; however, you must make it clear to him that this behavior is limited to the doll. He may not bite, hit, or harm the baby.

Pediatricians will bear witness to the fact that tiny babies *are* occasionally bitten by their eighteen-month-old sibling. One mother tells the story of her eighteen-month-old daughter dragging her three-day-old to her by its head. The baby was fine, but the story does illustrate the fact that the baby should not be left unattended with a preschooler in the house. One mother solved this problem by installing a dutch door to the baby's room. She could leave the top half open and lock the bottom half.

Every child will react to a new baby in his own way. The two-year-old may be very quiet and subdued, or he may be aggressive and demanding. He may start showing off and getting into mischief just to get your attention. His newly mastered toilet habits may give way to wetting his pants again. He may also insist on your feeding him again. You may feel dismayed at this, but try to understand the reason for his behavior and give him extra loving and comfort. Getting angry with him will only increase his feelings of exclusion and jealousy.

An older child may have more complex reactions than the preschool child. He may handle the new situation by ignoring you, or if he has a younger brother or sister (other than the baby) he may take his hostility out on the younger child by teasing him or encouraging him to get into trouble.

Involve your older child in a way that emphasizes his importance. "Baby Mark is crying; maybe a toy would make him happy. Could you pick one for him? He seems to like the toys you give him." Suggest giving the toys one at a time, and tell him to keep the toys away from the baby's face. Always emphasize the positive. Point out how the baby smiles when your older child comes into the room. "Look how baby Mark gets excited when he sees you." You will find this true. Babies seem to have a special interest in older siblings.

Avoid forcing the older child to kiss or hug the baby. Let the affection come naturally, with time. If the child has been allowed to express both positive and negative feelings without your telling him how he should feel—for example, "You should love your little brother" —you will be able to sit back and watch a truly genuine love develop.

One pediatrician suggests that it takes about six months for most children to adjust to a new family member. Most of the problems discussed here will gradually disappear as your older child becomes secure in the knowledge that he is a special person and that your love for him is unique and constant.

TAKING CARE OF YOURSELF

A newborn takes up a tremendous amount of your time. You will be aware of the needs of the other family members and will be concerned that everyone is happy and well cared for. You will feel great demands on your time and energy and may wind up allowing no time for yourself. It's often difficult to do, but you should set aside time for yourself. Do not feel you are being selfish. It's important for your well-being and the well-being of your family. If you are not rested, everyone will suffer. You will be less patient and happy. You may feel resentful. This will affect how you relate to your mate, baby, and other children.

Make time for you and your husband to be alone. Maintain your "coupleness." Many counselors advise getting out together alone on a weekly basis without the children. It's healthy to have a time when you can give full attention to one another without disruption from the baby and other children.

You must take care of yourself physically, too. Your scar will be shrinking more each day. You may notice hard scar tissue immediately under the incision. This is normal and will gradually soften. If there are small adhesive strips holding the incision together, do not be concerned if they fall off. Your doctor will probably have you leave the incision without a dressing, open to the air. *If your incision looks or feels different in any way* from how it did when you left the hospital, notify your doctor.

GET PLENTY OF REST

The day you come home from the hospital will be especially tiring. You should go to bed as soon as you can. Getting plenty of rest and sleep is essential for a fast recovery from surgery. Rest is also important if you are breastfeeding. Finding time to rest will take some planning, particularly if you have an older child or children at home.

Expect to feel tired both physically and mentally for some time after the birth of the baby. In addition to planning times to rest, you will have to use your available energy wisely. Organize your priorities, and don't overdo. A good guideline is to care only for yourself and the baby the first week you are home. If you have a child at home, spend relaxed time with him. Perhaps he can bring you story books to read and crawl into bed with you.

Consider staying in your robe or nightgown this first week. This will remind everyone that you are convalescing from major surgery and need lots of rest.

Keep some healthy snacks and beverages by your bedside. Bring your hospital tray home for this purpose. Some women enjoy keeping a good book or some needlepoint by the bed to help them relax. During the day, keep your baby next to your bed, along with diapers and other items you might need throughout the day. Keep a supply of plastic bags handy to use for disposing of dirty diapers.

Try to keep visitors away your first week at home. They invariably come just as you are about to take a nap. They stay too long and put undue pressure on you to have a tidy, clean house. Relatives who are anxious to see the newborn can be encouraged to do so at the hospital before you go home. Visitors and family too often cause unnecessary stress at an already stressful time. You will be recuperating from major surgery, and the entire family will be adjusting to a new family member. Decide before you come home from the hospital how you will handle unexpected guests.

HOUSEHOLD HELP

You will require full-time help at home the first week, and if you can get help for two weeks that's even better. If your mother or mother-in-law makes you feel nervous or inadequate, it is best to make other arrangements. Husbands are wonderful help if they can take time off from work to be with you and the baby. The person helping you should be responsible for the laundry, meals, marketing, and keeping the house tidy and running smoothly.

One mother, looking back on her experience, said "If I were to have another cesarean, John and I would hire help for a couple of weeks after surgery and once a week for a few weeks before, to take care of big cleaning jobs and any heavy work."[2]

THE SECOND WEEK

The second week you may begin to do light housekeeping chores with intermittent rest periods. For example, if you prepare breakfast, rest with your feet up for a while before doing the dishes. If you are feeling good, you may tend to overdo. Learn to recognize your body's signs of being tired. The secret is to *stop before you feel tired.* Be sure to accept all offers of help.

If you live in a two-story house, avoid trips up and down the stairs. Set up a place to change the baby both upstairs and downstairs. Also have a place downstairs where you can lie down to rest. Breast-feeding mothers may find it relaxing to lie down while feeding their babies.

THE THIRD WEEK

Once you are back to preparing meals,* you may find 4 to 6 P.M. to be the most trying time of the day. Colicky babies seem to get fussy during these hours. You and your toddler will be tired from the activities of the day. Your husband comes home. Your attention will be diverted to half a dozen different matters. To minimize this, plan simple meals that can be prepared in the morning. You might find a crock pot very useful. As a convalescing mother with a new baby, you will probably realize you will never get all the housework done in a day. However, if a messy house annoys you and your husband you will be concerned about keeping the house tidy. Try collecting all items that are out of place in a large basket periodically during the day or just before your husband gets home from work. Later, after dinner, or whenever it's convenient, put everything away. Get everyone to pitch in and help you. This method will make the housework much easier. (Some of these ideas may seem to be simple common sense, but sometimes it is easy to overlook simple solutions.)

Continue to nap during the day. Napping is very important because your sleep is being interrupted at night by the baby. Use your relaxation techniques so you can get the maximum benefit from your resting periods when you are not actually sleeping.

Avoid lifting for the first two weeks, to permit the incision to heal. Avoid even lifting the baby, initially. Have someone give the baby to you.

You may wonder how you are going to hold your other child on your lap with a sore abdomen. Try placing a pillow on your abdomen to protect it when holding your child. To avoid knees and feet in the abdomen, reach for your child before he climbs up on you and gently guide his approach. Gently remind the child that your abdomen is sore, too.

Your vaginal flow (lochia, or discharge of blood, mucus, and tissue from the uterus) will be decreasing and changing in color from red to brown to yellow-white to colorless. This flow lasts one to six weeks after birth. Use sanitary pads only, not tampons. If you notice an increase in vaginal flow (soaking more than two sanitary pads in half an hour), or if the flow was brown and suddenly turns bright red again, *tell your doctor*. Such a change usually indicates that you are overdoing and should go to bed and rest. As noted earlier, if you are passing large clots or if the discharge has a strong unpleasant odor, these are signs of a problem and should be reported. A temperature of 101° F or higher, or breasts that are red or feel hot or painful, should also be reported. It is normal to feel tired after a cesarean, but if you are feeling poorly and your appetite is poor over a period of time, tell your doctor.

FEEDING YOUR BABY

Breastfeeding your baby does not mean you cannot go out without your baby. There are several ways of handling such occasions. Some pediatricians suggest leaving formula for the baby to be fed while you are out. You may find that the baby will not take formula from you or take it if you are nearby because the baby smells your milk; however, many babies will take formula from someone else.

It is best to leave *your* milk to be given by your husband or a babysitter while you are out. Express, either by hand or with a pump, any milk left after each feeding, or express 2 ounces or so about one hour before feeding. It should be expressed into a plastic bottle, bag, or some other cold, sterile container (putting it through a dishwasher is sufficient sterilization). Cover it and label it with the date. The milk will remain usable up to six months in the freezer in your refrigerator and up to two years in a deep-freeze.

Tracy Hotchner, in her book *Pregnancy and Childbirth*, suggests introducing the baby to the person who will be giving the substitute feeding.[3] The person should stay for increasingly long periods of time but make no attempt to feed the baby the first few times. The first time you go away, plan to stay one to two hours and be within reach by phone. The person caring for the baby should try to feed the baby about half an hour before the baby's usual feeding time. Feeding before the baby gets really hungry makes it easier for him to cope with the bottle. The sitter should gently insert the nipple in a back-and-forth manner and stop if the baby gets too upset, trying again fifteen to twenty minutes later. Putting honey on the nipple may help, as well as using Nuk nipples, which are very much like human nipples. If the baby gets really upset, you may need to return and try again the following day. Some babies take longer than others to adjust to being bottle-fed.

Fathers enjoy the nice feelings associated with satisfying and

---

*We are not assuming that all women are or should be in charge of meals, but that role division is still usual, so we are dealing with current general practice.

soothing a hungry baby. Bottle-feeding can be shared equally between mother and father, as can be the responsibility for setting times for feedings.

Your eighteen-month-old child may also decide he wants a bottle again. Without comment, let him have a bottle *for all his liquid nourishment.* He will soon grow tired of drinking out of a bottle. If you are nursing, your older child will be fascinated. He may wish to taste the milk from your breast, too. If you are very casual about it and say "Sure," he will timidly take a sip and that will more than likely be the end of it.

RESUMING SEXUAL RELATIONS

Many cesarean mothers report that they did not feel interested in sex for a period of time after the baby was born. This is also not unusual for women who have experienced vaginal births. Much psychic and physical energy is required after the birth of a baby. There are nights of interrupted sleep, and many adjustments must be made by the entire family. Physical recovery from either form of childbirth takes a minimum of six weeks. Hormonal changes also account for a lack of interest in sex. Give yourself time and *credit* for coping with these enormous changes. If you have no desire for sex, do not be disturbed by this. It is quite normal, and with time your interest will return. Some women report it taking as long a six to nine months for their previous sexual interest to return. Generally, your doctor will give you the OK to resume sex at your six-week checkup.

Intercourse may not be comfortable for you at first, unless you use Vaseline or K-Y jelly for lubrication. When your hormonal levels return to their prepregnancy levels, this will no longer be necessary.

Some women feel physically unattractive after having babies because of their scars and big abdomens. If you have such feelings, it would probably be wise to start an exercise program to strengthen those abdominal muscles as soon as the doctor permits. Do not start without his approval.

Men are sometimes afraid that intercourse might hurt their wives. If this is the case, you might want to have your husband talk with the doctor. A comfortable position to try is with the woman on top.

Sometimes a weekend away from home, without the children and other pressures helps revive those old feelings. Don't worry, you will be functioning normally before long.

POSTPARTUM EXERCISE

If you have had a cesarean, you will probably feel anxious to get your figure back in shape. Not only have your abdominal muscles softened and stretched to accommodate the baby and the amniotic fluid, but the muscles have also been severed. Your abdomen is soft and sore and must have time to heal.

Most reconditioning literature for mothers who have just had a baby—the brochures you might pick up in the doctor's office—include "pelvic floor exercises." You will not need to do these, even if you have labored, because the baby was not pushed down through the vagina. You *will* want to do the exercises that strengthen the abdominal wall and that eventually firm your tummy once again.

It's natural to be in a big hurry to get back into form-fitting clothes again and to feel attractive doing so. However, you must wait until you are healed. A good indication as to when you are ready to begin exercises is when you can do them without feeling pain. It may hurt a little in the beginning, but if it hurts a lot, wait another week and try again.

Start your exercise program slowly and build up to the maximum amount gradually. You will not see results overnight. Be patient. if you expect to flatten your stomach, you will have to work at it over an extended period of time. Be religious about doing the exercises on a daily basis. The exercises will not harm your incision, and they will enhance your general good health.

At about three weeks after you are home from the hospital, you can begin to *gradually* do the following exercises:

1. Lie on the floor and hook your feet under the edge of your bed or any heavy piece of furniture that lends itself to this activity. Put your arms out straight in front of you. Now slowly sit up. Lie back down again, slowly rolling down vertebra by vertebra as you go. Later on, you will be able to do this without hooking your feet under something for support. However, you must make sure that you can do this properly by yourself. To do a situp properly, you should hold your tummy in tightly and begin to sit up, watching your tummy as you go. Go as far as you can go while still holding your tummy in. If you lose control of your tummy and it pops out (you can see this), then go back down. Eventually you will be able to get all the way up with your tummy firmly tucked in.

2. Lie flat on your back. Your arms should be at right angles flat on the floor. Bend your knees up, and lift your feet off the floor. Swing your bent knees toward the right and then the left, just twisting your body. Your shoulders and arms must stay flat on the floor.

3. Lie on your back, one leg bent with the foot flat on the floor. Raise the straight leg a few inches off the floor, hold to the count of three, then lower the leg and relax. Alternate legs and do it again. Later, when you have built up your muscles somewhat, do the same exercise, but this time raise your head and shoulders off the floor as you raise your leg.

4. Lie on the floor, on your back, with your knees bent. Hold your arms straight out in front of you. Now roll your head and shoulders up off the floor as far as you can. Relax slowly.

5. Lie on your back on the floor. Spread your feet wide apart, with your arms stretched to the sides. Raise your head as high as you can, and swing your right hand over to touch your right knee. Relax. Do the same thing on the other side.

6. Stand with your feet apart, arms stretched to the sky. Bend and touch your left toes with your right hand. Your left arm will swing backward. Your arms will be positioned like the wings of an airplane as it swoops toward the earth. Keep your legs straight and your head relaxed. Straighten up, and alternate sides. This exercise will strengthen your back as well as your abdominal muscles.

7. Stand with your feet apart. Hold your hands behind your neck. Keep your hips pointing straight ahead while you twist your upper body from side to side.

These exercises will be beneficial to you if you take them slowly. Once you have had your six-week checkup and obtain approval from your doctor, you can begin any exercise program you want.

PART V

Cesarean Options

CHAPTER FIFTEEN

Father-Attended Cesarean Birth

One of the most dramatic and controversial birth options that has arisen from the humanizing of cesarean delivery is the father's presence in the surgical suite, sharing in the birth event. As you examine some of the viewpoints set forth in this chapter by participants (both professional and nonprofessional) in father-attended cesarean births, you will have a better understanding of what the experience is like and what issues lead to the controversy.

Although progressive hospitals have recognized the benefits of the father-attended cesarean birth, other hospitals and many doctors still resist permitting fathers in the cesarean delivery suite. A primary objection voiced by doctors is simply that fathers have never been allowed in the operating room. It is a hospital rule—tradition.

Regarding traditions, Dr. Jack Klausen, an obstetrician who has performed numerous father-attended cesareans and is an outspoken advocate of the procedure, says

> To allow a father to attend his wife's cesarean childbirth breaks a long, hallowed tradition. I remember my first days in an operating room—the inner sanctum—where a dedicated team of medical professionals: surgeons, nurses, and technicians worked diligently to repair sick or broken bodies and to obtain the best possible outcome for the patient. To allow a layperson in this sacred place, in any role other than patient, was never considered nor tolerated.
>
> Like any tradition, the inviolate inner sanctum of the operating room went unquestioned for decades. "Professionals only"

was the inflexible rule. But this tradition, as any other, is wrong if it interferes with the well-being of a patient.

Of course, tradition is always well documented in hospital policies, making it even more difficult to question or change. Obviously, if something is written out as policy, it must be right.

The policy of barring fathers from the O.R. [operating room] reflects the expressed wishes of the health profession but does not consider the legitimate desire of a mother and father to be together to share the birth of their child, or the resulting benefits derived thereof.

Having a cesarean section is more than a surgical process; it is, after all the birth of a baby. For this reason I believe that anyone who observed the O.R. at the time of birth would conclude that the most important person in the room is the husband. With the father present, there is a feeling of completeness, particularly at that awesome moment of birth, when the couple becomes a family or adds a much cherished member to its family. It is popular to refer to what is happening psychologically and emotionally to the mother, father, and baby as they share the birth experience as "bonding." At that moment, I often feel philosophical. I feel better about where this baby is going. The family microcosm that I witness is unified and working together with love, compassion, and excitement.[1]

Considerations other than the inertia of tradition have stood in the way of the growth of father-attended cesareans. Dr. Klausen describes the fears expressed by some physicians:

Change in tradition usually starts with a few people questioning the unquestionable. When I began allowing the fathers in the operating room for a cesarean section, some of the arguments I heard from other doctors included [the following]:

- "Let a father in the O.R.? He'll pass out the first time he sees blood on the drapes."

- "A father in O.R.? Man, you've got a ready-made witness if anything goes wrong. You don't know this guy. How do you know you can trust him?"

- "I'd feel nervous. I couldn't relax if I had my patient's husband breathing down my neck."

- "If the father is in the O.R., I'd feel like if I smile or say something less than absolutely serious, he would feel I wasn't taking my job seriously."

Such fears are unfounded. To our knowledge, a father has never fainted or gone berserk in a cesarean surgical suite. To the contrary, his presence is calming to his wife and heightens the birth experience for all the participants, including the doctors and nurses. If anything out of the ordinary happens to a father, he can be quickly attended to by a circulating nurse with little distraction to others.

A trained father is not a distraction to the doctor; in fact, he can be a help by calming his wife. Many doctors have commented that having the father present ensures a more relaxed and thus a better patient. Again, Dr. Klausen agrees:

I consider the father-attended cesarean delivery, or, as I like to say, "the father-assisted cesarean delivery," as a further attempt by the medical profession to humanize the delivery of health care. As we heap more and more technology on people in the hospital, there is unfortunately a tendency to pay more attention to the machines monitoring the patient than to the patient herself. This fascination with machinery can leave a gap for the patient, who requires individual emotional reassurance. The father fills this gap in the father-assisted cesarean delivery. With a properly prepared father at the head of the table, where he can comfort his wife, our job becomes much easier and more proficient. This father support can only add to the technical knowledge and medical abilities of the doctors and nurses in maximizing the probability of a safe delivery and swift recovery.

My anesthesiologist often comments that with the husband present he uses much less of the tranquilizing medicines often needed to calm women as the surgery proceeds.

A feared increase in malpractice lawsuits has never materialized. Actually, there are probably fewer such lawsuits because of the rapport between the doctors and the parents. The husband has a firsthand opportunity to witness the hard work, expertise, and concern going into any emergency measures being taken by the medical team. One lawyer who is also a cesarean father commented,

People often sue doctors because they feel a particular doctor did not put forth his best effort in a given situation, or because they feel a doctor slighted them. A lawsuit is often a manifestation of an emotional phenomenon.

My strongest impression of the doctors during my wife's cesarean surgery was one of technical competence and immense skill—in a word, professionalism. I don't think my experience was unique in this respect.[2]

Proponents of this procedure feel that everyone involved benefits from the father's presence at the time of birth. Mothers get necessary emotional support during a frightening experience. Ordinarily, women do not complain as much about their physical difficulties following surgery as about their fears, feelings of alienation and loneliness, and anxieties about their babies. If the father is present, the mother is a happier patient.

Fathers benefit from being an important and integral part of the process. They are pleased and proud to have firsthand knowledge of what has happened in childbirth to pass on to their wives, family, and friends. A father enjoys the deep feeling of closeness that develops between him and his wife during childbirth and afterwards experiences the satisfaction that comes from knowing that his wife was happy with him and with the part he played in the drama of childbirth. And the father wants to see the miraculous moment of birth, a sight he will always carry in his memory and will often describe to his wife and children.

There is growing evidence that the way in which a new life is welcomed into this world has a bearing on the relationship between the parents and the child that extends through life. The father naturally wants to feel he has a close connection with the baby from the very beginning. He wants to be among the first to hear the baby's first cry, to hold him, love him, and share him with his wife. His fathering role can begin right there in the delivery room.

A benefit to the baby as well as the parents is the positive outlook stimulated by this childbirth experience. It enhances the likelihood that the parents will approach their nurturing roles and future pregnancies with a healthy mental attitude and confidence.

To realize these benefits, the prospective father must be properly prepared to attend the cesarean delivery. This means the father should take a cesarean childbirth class or obtain some instruction, along with accompanying visual aids, in a traditional natural childbirth class such as Lamaze or Bradley. He should read whatever he can about cesarean births and discuss the procedure with the obstetrician and pediatrician. He should try to visit the operating room sometime before the day of surgery to acquaint himself with the surroundings. If he has done all this, the father is unlikely to misunderstand what he sees or hears during the surgery. In reality, a cesarean father is so occupied with his wife and baby during the operation that he does not pay much attention to the doctors. If an emergency should arise, he may be asked to leave, but chances are he will be allowed to stay. The decision is up to the doctor. Proper preparation thus minimizes fears that have been expressed by some doctors and will permit all concerned to benefit from the father's presence. Dr. Klausen's experience confirms this:

> We doctors are subject to the same types of fears and worries as everyone else. Because of the enormity of our responsibility, these fears are often magnified. We really do want what is best for our patients. We don't always agree on what that may be. Many doctors feel that they *always* know what is best for their patient. However, more and more of us are listening to the patient's desires and needs, and in doing so are learning some valuable lessons while dispelling some old ideas. Nowhere has this trend been more evident than with respect to father-attended cesarean birth. If the skeptics could only see what I have seen at these deliveries, I believe their uneasiness and doubts would dissipate.

Obstetricians are not the only members of the surgical team who appreciate the benefits of a father-attended cesarean birth.

Dr. Stephen Jackson, an anesthesiologist at Good Samaritan Hospital in San Jose, California, addressing the Cesarean Birth Council, says,

> Reemphasizing humanism in medicine is, I believe, today's greatest challenge for the modern-day physician. The basic tenets of humanistic medicine (1) encourage people to actively assume responsibility for maintenance of their own physical and psychological well-being, and (2) utilize medical experiences as creative opportunities for psychological growth. A significant development in this field has involved the introduction of paternal participation with labor and vaginal delivery. A logical extension of this now well-accepted humanistic concept is the presence of the father in the cesarean-delivery operating room. Indeed, the humanistic physician should encourage and facilitate the desire of expectant parents to share their child's birth.
>
> The bonding of the family unit from the moment of birth is the most personally gratifying experience in my medical practice. The touching of hands, the reassuring smiles, the shared excite-

ment, the loving verbiages, the visual messages of caring, the crescendo of psychological optimism and support, the gleeful utterances of the moment of birth—these are but part of the transcendental moments of the universal joys of parenthood that are possible only in the setting of a sharing couple.

Indeed, the task of the anesthetist is eased by the father's presence in the operating room before, during and after the cesarean delivery of a mother with a regional (spinal, lumbar epidural, or caudal) anesthetic. Maternal anxiety is significantly allayed and her apprehension dissipated. It is much easier to administer the anesthetic when the father holds the mother in position. I have noted a significant decrease in the incidence of nausea and vomiting as well as of a number of various other subjective symptoms such as dizziness, light-headedness, and difficulty in breathing. With the father attending to the majority of the mother's psychological needs, the anesthetist is able to expend more of his energies in providing the mother and her fetus with the most advantageous physiological environment.[3]

The pediatrician is on hand for the delivery, but is not directly involved with the surgery, which puts him (or her) in a unique position to direct his attention to the dynamics of the birth experience. Dr. Trianto, a pediatrician, observes, "Even the doctors benefit from observing firsthand what this delivery means to the entire family." And, in regard to the newborn, "Infants get the benefit of more contented and closer parents, and who knows what that may mean in their future."[4]

A cesarean delivery is one of the few surgical procedures in which a doctor can immediately see joy in others resulting from his work. It is a happy experience—just ask a doctor who has performed, or been involved in, a father-shared cesarean.

FROM A FATHER'S PERSPECTIVE

The experience as seen through the eyes of a father can be very exciting. The following is a random collection of stories and reflections on a shared cesarean delivery from some fathers and mothers. We have included them to provide you participants' views of this joyous birth option.[5]

Our first story is a touching and complete account of a father-attended cesarean birth, related by Harry Leff, a cesarean father. We think you will enjoy his story.

When I reflect on the birth of my second daughter, Jocelyn Cara, suddenly every detail flashes before me. If someone had told me that someday I'd not only be witness to the birth of my child but be present during major surgery, I'd have questioned their sanity. But suddenly there I was in hospital greens, all scrubbed up and ready to go.

I guess I should start this story from the beginning. Actually this story came close to not being at all. After the birth of our first daughter Megan Renee, under the conditions of an emergency cesarean section, my wife was convinced she would never go through that again. There we were, our Lamaze certificate in hand, ready to partake in the joy of natural childbirth, when after seventeen hours of labor the world began crumbling around us. Suddenly I was asked to leave the labor room, with no real explanation as to why my wife, who was experiencing great pain due to back labor [pain in low back rather than abdomen] was rushed to x-ray. A few minutes later, the doctor told me they were going to do an emergency C-section [cesarean]. This nightmare [went] on and on. Fortunately, mother, daughter, and father came through it all right.

It took us about $2^1/2$ years to muster the courage to try again. Of course, this time we knew the birth would have to be a repeat cesarean. I give my wife a lot of credit. I don't think I would have willingly gone through that operation again.

Suddenly it happened—we were pregnant! Hooray for us! But not really. For we knew at the end of the long nine months ahead lay a week of pure hell.

It was shortly after our confirmation of pregnancy that my wife began looking for an obstetrician. It was the doctor she chose who first planted the seed in Leslie's mind that dear old Dad could share "Hell Week" and actually be present during the surgery. All we had to do was attend some classes that would train us in such necessary techniques as which way Daddy should fall during surgery and "all babies look that way when they are first born."

After some thought, I came to a decision. I would go to the classes but would not make any commitment on whether or not to participate in the surgery.

Our first class reminded me of the first day of school. Everyone was very still and quiet. We all tried to sit in the back of the room, but with only four couples that was pretty hard. The classes dealt with two basic themes. The first one was very technical, dealing with the surgical procedure and related information, while the second unveiled the psychological aspect of cesarean birth.

It was the latter that I found most interesting. I learned, among other things, that some women develop a sense of inadequacy, as if they had failed as women for not being able to deliver the "natural way." My own wife disclosed some inner feelings that I never knew before. The discussions really broke down some deep hidden emotional barriers that could potentially obstruct the joy of childbirth.

Already things were looking better for us both. We were both more relaxed and starting to enjoy the pregnancy stage, as we had during our first. The usual scenes were taking place. We painted the baby's room, started organizing the baby clothes, and began the lengthy process of picking a name. And, to make it even better, Leslie was having a terrific, care-free pregnancy. She had never been so happy and healthy in all her life.

Now it was December, the month things were beginning to take form. I had pretty much decided to be in the operating room during the delivery but I was quick to qualify it by saying I would hold Leslie's hand but not look at anything. That was acceptable to her. Finally, after much harassing and pestering, the doctor told us the baby would be born on January 10 at 2 P.M. My first reaction to this news was to think how I would organize a betting pool at work on which day the baby would be born. Of course, I would get the first pick. Things were moving along nicely. Then suddenly it was January 9, or I guess you could call it Jocelyn Eve. Leslie got Megan off to bed. I built a fire and poured us both a glass of wine. It was a beautiful evening, one that brought us even closer together.

It was incredible how well we both slept. Maybe it was the wine. But now it was January 10, and the alarm went off about 7 A.M. I looked outside the window. It was pouring rain. While Leslie was getting showered and dressed, I got Megan ready for nursery school. Megan knew Mommy was going to the hospital today to have a "brother sister," as she would put it.

Megan and I had breakfast alone together, as Mommy was not supposed to eat anything. Now it was about 9. We had to drop Megan off at school and be at the hospital by 10 to check in.

Unlike the hurried atmosphere of checking into the hospital when your wife's pains are three minutes apart, this time was very relaxed for us both. I kept looking at Leslie and thinking,

"When is this happy, care-free façade going to crack? How could anyone about to face surgery be so cheerful?" But I am glad to report she never lost one ounce of that optimism during her entire hospital stay. She was truly an example of positive thinking. Anyway, we sat in the lobby of the hospital for a few minutes until a rather pleasant middle-aged lady asked us to follow her to the admitting office. Here we answered the usual questions for the hospital records and were given some personal items for Leslie to take to her room.

It was then that we met Pat and Arnie. Pat and Leslie were both patients of Dr. S. and had met in his office. As it turned out, Pat's surgery was scheduled for 1 P.M. to be followed by Leslie's at 2. Needless to say, in the next few days we became pretty good friends.

Now it was time to go to our room. Pat and Arnie were already there. Leslie was shown the bathroom, where she could change into a hospital gown. While she was out, Arnie and I began to talk. He could not believe I was going to watch my wife's surgery. Arnie was a nervous wreck. He tried to cover up his nervousness but was failing poorly.

Leslie came out of the bathroom in her hospital gown and got into bed. A nurse came in to check her blood pressure, temperature, and so on. She said the doctors would be in shortly. The first to arrive was our obstetrician. Since both patients were his, he gave the pitch once for both to hear. He then reiterated Pat's desire to be put completely under during her surgery. He turned, looked at me, and said, "Well, you ready to go?" It is amazing how fear can quickly contract every muscle in your body. Anyway, I smiled at him and nodded. He next asked Leslie if she had any questions. She replied no, and off he went.

We had brought along a deck of cards to help pass the time. We got in a few hands of gin before the nurse returned to prep Leslie. I was asked to leave. To this day, Leslie swears the prepping is worse than the surgery. Upon completion of the task, the nurse stepped out and told me I could go back in. The look on Leslie's face was reminiscent of someone stepping on a roller coaster for the first time. Among other things, they put a tight pair of elastic stockings on her to prevent blood pressure from dropping—something we had covered in class. Arnie and Pat were full of questions. It was then that we really felt good about the training we had received.

The next person to enter the room was a very special man,

our anesthesiologist. He explained to us the type of anesthesia he would use and what effects to expect. He was to later be a big factor in making this birth an enjoyable one.

Time was passing very quickly. Nurses were buzzing around like bees in a hive, straightening up beds, checking blood pressures, and so on. Now it was time for Pat to leave. You could tell both she and Arnie were nervous. It was almost sad. Pat went one way, Arnie went the other. I could see Arnie down the hall, doing the stereotyped pacing bit that all fathers are supposed to do. I really felt sorry for him.

A short time later, twenty minutes or so, Arnie came in with a giant smile on his face: "It's a boy!" We were real happy for them. Now it was our turn.

An orderly brought in a gurney and helped Leslie get on it. I kissed her and said, "See you in a little while." I was sure she was going to crack, but she held up well. A few minutes later, a nurse came into the room with a stack of ugly, wrinkled, but clean hospital "greens." She told me it was time to get dressed. I was not too nervous, even though it was then I discovered the hole in the pants was not for your head. Oh, well, we all make mistakes.

Now time was getting close. I had remembered from class that it would be approximately fifteen minutes from the time Leslie left to the time they would come for me. I stared at the clock. Fifteen minutes went by, but I was still there. Now twenty, then thirty. All I could think about was [that] something had gone wrong. I corraled a nurse and informed her of my plight. She said she would check. It seems they were a little slow in cleaning up the operating room after Pat's surgery. What a horrible picture that conjured up in my mind!

While standing in the hall waiting, I will never forget overhearing two nurses converse about that patient who was waiting to go into the operating room. They both agreed they had never seen anyone so well prepared mentally for surgery. I knew they meant Leslie. I was so proud of her. There was no way I would fall apart during the surgery now. I was inspired.

Finally, after an eternal forty-five minutes, a smiling nurse came for me. She directed me to an area where there were some sinks. I was handed a little package containing a scrub brush filled with soap and instructed to scrub up to my elbows for five minutes. No cheating. It is normally ten, but I had already scrubbed for five at the nurses' station.

What a trip! At the sinks behind me were our obstetrician

and his assistant surgeon. Next to me was our pediatrician, whom I had never met.

After passing inspection, I was told to wait outside until the doctors had finished prepping Leslie and had administered the anesthesia. Now it was time to go in.

My first thought upon entering the operating room was "I must be in the wrong place." This did not even come close to the operating rooms I have seen on TV. The walls were a nice, bright yellow, and it just did not have that cold sterile feel I had expected. The funniest part was when I noticed the doctor's tools were lying on top of a Sears Craftsman tool chest. I could not believe it. I was not sure at that point if Leslie was having a baby or getting a tune-up.

I was led over to a stool at the head of the table, where I was to sit. To my right was the anesthesiologist, and between us was Leslie's head. That is all I could see. Her head and left arm. The anesthesia screen blocked the rest from view.

The anesthesiologist asked Leslie how she felt. Her reply was "A little dizzy." Sure enough, her blood pressure had dropped. The anesthesiologist ordered a nurse to place a folded-up sheet under her right side. This did the trick. It was then that I learned who really runs the operating room. When the obstetrician noticed Leslie was tilted, he grumbled, "Get this sheet out of here." The anesthesiologist replied, "It stays." He then explained the problem, and the obstetrician retreated.

Now it begins. Leslie felt a slight sensation at the beginning. She was given some nitrous oxide (laughing gas). There she was, sprawled across the table laughing her head off. The surgeon then suggested that the anesthesiologist pass it around so we could all have a good time. But finally Leslie calmed down. Every time the anesthesiologist gave her something, he also turned to me to say what effect the drug would have. For example, once he cautioned me that a certain drug could cause a temporary lapse of memory so I should not be alarmed if Leslie asked the same question repeatedly. His concern for me really made the occasion something special. I was part of the birth, not just an outsider.

About seven or eight minutes had passed when the doctor said, "Daddy, stand up, here comes the baby." I took a deep breath and stood. Suddenly a head covered with black hair appeared. I narrated this to Leslie; she could not believe it, as our first, Megan, was a baldy. Next came the shoulders and voila!—a baby girl! Congratulations came from everyone. Leslie began to cry. The doctor inquired why she was crying, concerned that it was from pain and not happiness. Our obstetrician showed Leslie the baby and quickly handed her to our pediatrician. I sat back on my stool. Leslie held my hand tightly.

From where I sat, I could see the pediatrician busily examining Jocelyn. Oh yes, we had announced her name to everyone there. No more than two minutes had passed when the pediatrician turned to me and said, "Hey, Daddy, you want to watch?" By now I was ready to watch anything and everything. I was escorted to his work area. I watched for about thirty seconds, and then he bundled Jocelyn up in his arms, moved toward me, and said, "Here is your daughter." It was the heaviest 8 pounds, $1^1/_2$ ounces, I had ever held. Boy, was it great! Jocelyn and I were escorted to Mommy. Leslie touched her toes and again began to cry. I wish that moment could have lasted forever. Jocelyn was beautiful. No doubt about it.

I finally had to surrender Jocelyn to a nurse. I did so and again sat down. Another nurse called me over to another table to sign some papers stating that I had witnessed the birth and that mother's and baby's identification numbers were the same. Now it was back to my stool again. I was waiting for someone to say "Time to go" to me. That is what we were led to believe in class. After the baby was born, Daddy would leave the baby—but no one asked me to leave. The obstetrician must have sensed that I was in total control of myself. He even insisted I stand and watch a new closing technique. It resembled staples.

I know that the doctors, nurses, and scrub technicians that had taken part in the delivery have probably been through this hundreds of times, but I swear, they were almost as excited as Leslie and I.

Now it was over. The whole thing took only twenty-two minutes. I gave Leslie a kiss and told her I would see her after she got out of recovery. In my excitement, I forgot to thank everyone, but made up for it by later writing a letter to the hospital chief administrator commending his staff.

Earlier I mentioned how I felt sorry for Arnie. Let me elaborate. I walked out from the operating room area, still in my greens, and over to the nursery. Arnie was full of questions: "Was it bloody? What was it like?" and so on, and on. He was really jealous.

To witness the birth of your child has got to be one of the high points of your life. After missing out on our first, this one more than made up for it.

This story really has no end. Even as I write, Jocelyn is ten months old, crawling up my leg and trying to teethe on the paper. It really perks me up when I look at her and think back to her birthday. I hope all fathers who have the opportunity do not let it pass by. I am glad I didn't.

Each couple's experience is unique to them. However, they all share the common aspects of awe, joy, and closeness.

One father describes the powerful family bonding that can be created by shared cesarean birth:

I will always have the picture in my head of our baby being born. They asked me if I wanted to stand up—I was sitting during the operation—so I stood up. I saw the head appear. I heard those first, wet-sounding cries. I saw the doctors cleaning and suctioning him out, and then the rest of his body was born. As soon as I saw that he was a boy baby, he was Matt. That was the name we had picked out.

When he was cleaned up, the doctor brought him over to us, and I got to hold him. My wife got to feel his little leg and foot and touch him. He became a person for us right then.

Another father told us,

It was great to see my baby being born. It was exciting. I was telling Celia what I saw and what was happening at different times, and she was smiling.

The only complaint I had was that I couldn't see as much as I wanted to. When the doctors told me I could stand up, they were about to bring the baby out, I was so excited I could hardly talk. I saw his head first, and he had a kind of tissue all over his face. The doctors started suctioning. He didn't start crying right away. He reminded me of a little rubber doll. They pulled and pulled, and finally he was out. He was a beautiful boy. He was just big and healthy and fine. The experience was everything we had expected it to be.

Another father reacted thus:

When it got to the point where they were ready to take the baby, I was invited to stand up and watch. I was a little afraid, because I had never seen surgery before, but I stood up. It wasn't at all shocking. Yes, there was blood, but you are in a state of mind that [you know] you're not there to see the blood, you're there to see the child being born. When I think about the whole thing, I don't think about anything that was gruesome or bloody. I remember the first thing that happened was the head popped out. Then the shoulders came out, and then the doctor pulled her out and said, "You've got a nice little girl here." I told him she was Teresa, and he said "That's a pretty name." My wife and I were talking, and everyone was congratulating themselves. The nurses were smiling and happy. The pediatrician had the baby, and I guess he could see nothing was wrong so, to my surprise, he asked me to watch the baby getting her physical. Then within three or four minutes he said, "Here," and gave me the baby. This was a total shock, because I didn't get to hold my first daughter until she was about four days old, but here I'm holding this baby that's part of my wife and myself that's only three or four minutes old. I took her over to my wife and watched her eyes as she touched the baby's foot. I think my excitement and our joy spread around the whole operating room. Everyone was excited. Everyone was happy.

Another father also felt he had participated in a rare and beautiful experience. He quickly jotted down his impressions of the birth before leaving the hospital. He wanted to do this while everything was fresh in his mind and he was still feeling the excitement of the day. These are his notes:

Momentary confusion upon entering operating room. Green everywhere. People busy, but relaxed. Very professional. Anesthesiologist directs me to my stool. My head is right next to Kathy's. She has a green plastic mask on and a green cap. I didn't expect the mask. Anesthesiologist pulls back the drape covering Kathy so I could hold her arm. I occasionally push a piece of her hair back from her face that has come out of her cap. Anesthesiologist busy taking notes and monitoring blood pressure. IV's and tubes everywhere. Music playing. Soft. Very little conversation. I am surprised at how little verbal communication is necessary for the surgeons to work. Pediatrician waiting to receive baby. Nurses have warmed some blankets to receive the baby. Someone shows them to Kathy. Kathy wide awake. "How are you feeling?" "Excited." "Did you sleep well?" "Yes." "Did you?" "Yes." We talk with the supervising nurse about names we have selected for the baby depending on if it is a girl or a boy. I can't see much over the screen that is between Kathy's head and the doctors operating. Excitement intensifies. I look around. Anesthesiologist tells Kathy she has a good spinal block. Kathy's head is on a pillow. She feels no pain re: surgery. Here comes the baby. Anesthesiologist tells me I can peek over the screen. I see the baby's head. Kathy asks about hair color. Looks to me like dark hair. Baby is out. Very fast. Kind of gooey and bluish, and perfectly formed. I announce it's a girl. The doctor sticks his head over the screen and tells Kathy, "She's a big baby and just fine!" The umbilical cord is cut. Baby is put into warm blankets and taken to the warmer. Pediatrician takes over the baby. I sign form witnessing the birth! Pediatrician examines the baby. He then brings her over for Kathy to see. Kathy is smiling and happy. Baby is taken out of surgical suite. Kathy is going to be put to sleep. I say goodbye and leave with the nurse. I go to the nursery and watch the pediatrician weigh the baby. He holds up eight fingers, then three. She weighs 8 pounds, 3 ounces. she is big and chubby and pink and beautiful. Nurse brings me coffee, and I just watch for one half hour. The doctor comes out of the surgical suite. Everyone is pleased with the operation. Excited. Super great experience.

FROM A MOTHER'S PERSPECTIVE

Mothers who experienced cesarean childbirth before the time when fathers were allowed in the operating room, and who later had a father-attended cesarean can hardly believe the difference in the birth experience. Each story is unique but shares on common characteristic with all others—happiness.

Our first story from the mother's perspective is actually three stories: an emergency cesarean, a planned cesarean without the father present, and a father-attended cesarean. The contrasts among these birth experiences demonstrate the advantages of this latter option in a clear, self-explanatory fashion.

December 13, 1970. I have started labor with my first baby at twenty-four years of age. I have had a healthy pregnancy and am expecting a normal childbirth. After thirty-five hours of unsuccessful labor, I still have not given birth. I am drugged, but I understand that something has gone wrong. No one speaks to me. I can endure the pain no longer. I begin to scream hysterically, unceasingly. A kind but commanding voice says, "Karen." It's as though I have been slapped in the face. I stop screaming. (Later I was told that I never became hysterical and no one spoke my name. It must have all happened in my subconscious mind). I feel myself being pushed down the hall at a rapid pace. An intern appears at my head and tells me a cesarean section must be performed. Do I give my permission? Yes. Anything. Save my baby. Save me.

John, out in the waiting room where he has spent the night, is in a state of fatigue from lack of sleep and worrying. "What in God's name is taking so long? Have they forgotten I'm here? Why doesn't anybody tell me what is going on?"

Finally the doctor comes out to the waiting room. "I can see the baby's head now, but Karen's bone structure is too small, and her tail bone curves inward, blocking the baby's passage. I would have to pull hard to bring the baby out, and I am afraid of damaging her spine or injuring the baby." Of course, John signed the papers authorizing the doctor to perform a cesarean.

Surgery is about to begin. The doctor is at my head. It is the first time in hours that I am aware of his presence. I am so relieved to see him. He asks me if I want the incision to be in the regular direction (horizontal), or do I want it to be vertical in the same place as an earlier scar. My heart leaps for joy. I must not be going to die. That is not a question you ask a dying person. "I don't care about that," I tell him. I am going to live!

Finally a son is born. The doctor brings him out for John to see. He tells John that I am going to be fine. John cries and laughs. "He looks pretty beat up."

"Well," counters the doctor, "He looks a hell of a lot better than you do. Go home and get some sleep."

John looks down at his crumpled suit that he had slept in. He feels his thirty-six-hour growth of whiskers. "You're right," he grins, "but if you don't think I would frighten my wife, I would like to see her."

July 1, 1973. I am checked into the hospital to have my cesarean, the second child we want so much. Since my first baby was born, we have moved and I have another obstetrician and another hospital. I know this experience is going to be easier than the previous time, but I am nonetheless very frightened. Surgery begins, and again I am looking for some assurance that all is going well. Again, I see no one, and no one speaks to me. Then a nurse walks into my range of vision. She walks up to the wall, leans against it, crosses her legs, folds her arms, yawns, and stands there.

It feels good to see a human being, something I can recognize among all the shining metal apparatus. My eyes rivet on her face for a reading. She looks disinterested, almost bored. Good sign. Everything must be going well. I watch her face during the whole procedure for any change of expression that might indicate that some problem had occurred in surgery. None. I never saw her again, and she will never know she made a difficult time for a surgery patient somewhat easier by just standing and looking as though she was having the dullest time of her life. The doctor announces I have a healthy baby girl. I feel a surge of joy. It is short-lived. I am told I am going to be put to sleep. Good.

February 24, 1977. The long-awaited day has arrived. We are prepared this time. John will be with me for the birth of our baby. Surgery is scheduled for 8 A.M. I experience a bad case of butterflies minutes prior to surgery, which subside as soon as John joins me and the procedure is under way. Fear gives way to excitement. It is catching. John and the surgical team are smiling and talking. I am very conscious of the details of everything going on around me. The walls are yellow. There is soft music playing in the background. The nurses are preparing warm blankets to receive our baby. My senses are at a peak in anticipation of the momentous event about to take place. Sarah is born. John is invited to peek over the screen. I watch John's face as he witnesses the birth. It is a thrilling picture of amazement and joy. He holds my hand tighter and tighter. The baby is cleaned and in minutes brought to us—the happiest moment of all! Instead of feeling left out, I feel like the center of attention, like a proud mother, loved wife, and star patient. I have experienced childbirth in a new way and found it to be a pinnacle in emotional reward. It was a wonderful experience in sharing. And, even though I did not see my baby at the moment of birth, to see my husband's face as he witnessed it was a marvelous alternative and something I will always remember.

Another mother told us,

The biggest difference in this cesarean was having my husband in the delivery room with me and knowing what was going to happen before it happened. I wasn't just left out in the dark not knowing what was going to happen next. With Tony with me, I wasn't afraid. I didn't feel as though I was just in a butcher shop or something, you know. During surgery, I watched Tony's face, and listened to him talk. He would crack jokes and try and make me laugh, but I didn't want to laugh, because I was afraid the doctor would cut something he shouldn't.

Similarly, another mother described her feelings thus:

Having this cesarean with my husband with me is something I will never forget. It was joyous. I know my husband was nervous. I could tell when he was talking to me, telling me what was going on. He sounded nervous, but it was wonderful having him there. He was my lifeline at all times. We held hands, and he talked gently to me. When the baby was about to be born, the doctor told him to stand up. He did, still holding my hand, and said, "Oh, my God, look at all that black hair!" Knowing he was there for me and sharing the birth of our baby was a high point in my life. It was beautiful. It's something I will never forget.

Still another mother said,

I was afraid to have the spinal. This was the part I feared most. The doctor on my first cesarean had quite a bit of trouble giving me the spinal and finally lost patience with me. Also, I had talked to a girl whose spinal had been very painful. I was also worried that if the spinal did not go well my husband would not be allowed in. Happily, all my worrying was unnecessary because my spinal was fast and I didn't feel any pain. I'm sure the fact that I was prepared and cooperative made the difference. I experienced a few moments of slight nausea, which passed quickly.

Finally my husband was allowed in. What a relief to have him with me. I was never so glad to see him in my whole life. He sat down by my head and held my hand. It seemed like it took forever until the doctors reached my baby. Then someone said something about the baby coming, and Steve was standing, saying, "It's a boy. It's a boy!" I felt a surge of joy! Steve stayed at my side, and after the pediatrician checked the baby over he was brought to us. The baby was wrapped in blankets so I couldn't see his body, but someone took my hand and placed it on his foot. I never felt anything so soft and warm. Steve held him for a few minutes, and then he was taken back to the warmer. I wish we could have kept him longer because as the operation progressed I felt worse, and I know if the baby was with me I would have focused my attention on him instead of myself. I wasn't in real pain, but I felt very uncomfortable. I didn't want to be put out. I wanted to maintain as much control as possible, so I appreciated not having anything in the form of drugs forced on me. Even though I hurt, I felt proud of myself. I think Steve was surprised that his wife, who faints over a sliver in her thumb, could go through major surgery so easily. Two facts made for such a happy birth and speedy recovery—having my husband with me and having some knowledge about cesareans. Both of us now know that a cesarean birth can be a wonderful experience.

If it is your preference, you too, as a couple, can share the birth of your new baby.

CHAPTER SIXTEEN

Vaginal Birth After a Cesarean

"Once a cesarean, always a cesarean." Who hasn't heard this old saying? This dictum was pronounced by Dr. Edwin B. Cragin in 1916, and it became the general rule. The vast majority of obstetricians practicing in this country still abide by Dr. Cragin's adage. Cesarean mothers have always assumed that if they had their first baby by cesarean that all subsequent babies had to be delivered in the same fashion. Considering that recent figures show 98.9% of all women with a previous cesarean deliver surgically in subsequent pregnancies, it was a safe assumption.[1]

However, on February 25, 1985, 69 years after Dr. Cragin's pronouncement, Dr. Luella Klein, president of the American College of Obstetrics and Gynecology, announced at a news conference, that the long held medical doctrine of "once a cesarean, always a cesarean" is no longer true. According to Dr. Klein, 50% to 80% of the women who have had cesareans can deliver vaginally as long as they do not have what is known as a "classical" incision from their prior cesarean.

WHAT HAS BROUGHT ABOUT THIS CHANGE OF THOUGHT?

The main objection to a vaginal delivery after a cesarean has been fear of uterine rupture during labor that would result in loss of blood and seriously endanger the life of the fetus and mother. However, that argument has lost its validity according to the results of recent studies that show that vaginal birth after a cesarean (VBAC) has minimal risk. Dr. Klein states, "Although this rupture can occur, we have found that it is rarely catastrophic, as long as we have modern fetal monitoring, obstetrical support services and anesthesia, the mother's health and safety along with her infant's are protected.''

Because the risks of a cesarean are so low, we sometimes forget that they do exist. With a cesarean there is an increased risk of mortality, morbidity, and blood loss as compared to a normal birth. The medical costs are considerably higher and the hospital stay is longer. Feelings of diminished self-worth and failure also frequently accompany cesarean delivery, as discussed elsewhere in this book. Recovery is more difficult and lengthy than with a vaginal birth. When you return home, your body has to rebound from major surgery, which is always doubly difficult with a new baby.

Another significant benefit from allowing a trial of labor is that you know that the fetus has reached the maximum obtainable maturity when it is born.

ARE YOU A CANDIDATE FOR A VBAC?

Unfortunately, not every cesarean mother who desires a VBAC is a candidate for a trial of labor. There are criteria and guidelines to determine whether you could safely and successfully undertake a trial of labor.

A very crucial factor is the type of uterine incision the mother had previously. This is the incision on the uterus, not on the outer skin. Women considered for a trial of labor must have a low transverse incision, which means a horizontal incision in the lower part of the uterus.

The significance of the type of incision is that doctors are concerned about the danger of uterine rupture—that is, a hole, a partial separation, or the presence of a ''window'' in the scar tissue. This is not very serious. What is feared is a ''catastrophic rupture,'' which completely tears the scar tissue apart, expelling the baby out of the uterus into the abdominal cavity. This is usually fatal for the baby. The mother usually suffers from hemorrhage and shock. If the bleeding is uncontrollable, a hysterectomy is mandatory to save the woman's life. However, if the woman has had a low-segment transverse scar, she is unlikely to have a ''catastrophic rupture.'' Most reports state that uterine rupture incidences for low transverse incisions are between 0.25 and 0.5 percent. Most importantly, no maternal deaths have occurred in reported trials of labor.

Besides the type of incision, other factors govern whether or not a woman is a good candidate for a VBAC. Many doctors exclude women who have had more than one cesarean. Some doctors exclude women whose first cesarean was for a ''recurring indication.'' Cephalopelvic disproportion, in which the baby's head is too big to fit through the pelvis or birth canal, is considered to be a recurrent indication by most physicians. However, there is recent evidence that women who have had primary cesareans for this indication and who labor with a subsequent baby have a greater than 60 percent incidence of delivering vaginally.[2]

Indications such as breech position, placenta previa or abruptio, fetal distress, toxemia, and "failure of labor to progress" are considered by many doctors as unlikely to recur.

Some doctors think it is important that the mother have had one vaginal delivery before her cesarean and that she was free from postpartum infection with any cesarean delivery. They believe that infection in the uterus weakens the scar tissue.

Another criterion for trial labor is that the baby's head be "head first" down the pelvis (vertex presentation) at the onset of labor. The course of labor must be normal, and descent through the pelvis, as well as dilatation of the cervix, must progress at a normal rate. Also, most doctors consider a woman with a chronic disease such as diabetes a poor candidate for a VBAC.

You must be in good health and have a normal pregnancy. The presence of twins is a contraindication for a VBAC, as is a very large baby. The maximum fetus size for a VBAC is considered to be 4000 grams—about nine pounds. You must also understand that the trial of labor may end in a cesarean and that pain relievers may be limited during labor to better enable your doctor to determine whether there has been a uterine rupture.

Your obstetrician must consider the safety and practicality of a VBAC. You and your doctor must have access to a hospital that can re spond at any time to an obstetric emergency within thirty minutes, including 24-hour blood banking and anesthesia coverage. This should not prove to be a major deterrent to performing VBAC's as any hospital which admits patients for childbirth should have such facilities. After all, emergencies can arise with any delivery, and all first deliveries are, to some extent, trials of labor.

In an article discussing VBAC's the *American Journal of Obstetrics and Gynecology* addressed this point:

"The principal cry against [VBAC's] is that not all hospitals are equipped with adequate anesthesia or blood banks to handle the rare case of fetal distress or maternal hemorrhage that may accompany a ruptured uterus. If this is true, such a hospital should not be handling any obstetric cases, because acute fetal distress from an umbilical cord prolapse is a much more frequent event than fetal distress from a ruptured previous scar. Maternal hemorrhage from placenta previa or abruptia placentae is a much more frequent catastrophe than maternal hemorrhage from a ruptured uterus."[3]

In sum, if your hospital is not equipped to accommodate a VBAC, it should not be admitting patients for childbirth at all.

The practice of defensive medicine, i.e., avoidance of malpractice suits, by many physicians may impede the widespread acceptance by doctors of VBAC's.

Legal Concerns Regarding VBAC's

Obstetricians are justifiably concerned that they will be defendants in a malpractice suit if the result of pregnancy is anything other than a healthy, normal infant and mother. Realistically, but perhaps unfairly, perfection has become the expected standard. Any lesser result in the absence of the obstetrician doing all that is humanly possible (e.g. a cesarean section), is an invitation to litigation.

The explosion of malpractice litigation in the obstetrical field, coincident with tremendous strides in the safety and comfort of childbirth and childbirth experiences is one of the ironies of our litigious society. Indeed, it seems that the very low incidence of maternal and infant mortality have raised the expectations of prospective parents to such a high level that the natural conclusion in the event of a less than perfect result is that someone committed an error in judgment and/or execution. That someone is, of course, the obstetrician.

Dr. Eugene C. Sandberg, writing recently in the *American Journal of Obstetrics and Gynecology* commented:

"It is assumed without serious questioning (or thought) that this mantle of indestructibility (the low maternal mortality rate) encompasses the fetus and the neonate as well, that birth is a trivial event for the offspring. Few individuals associated with the pregnant woman seem aware of or give significant thought to the fact that perils still exist in pregnancy or that the potential for disaster is ever present. Everyone within range of the pregnant woman throughout her pregnancy anticipates (and reinforces the patient's anticipation of) happiness, joy, and fulfillment. In other words, success and a good result (a perfect baby) are to be expected and are the natural sequelae to becoming pregnant."

Against this background of high expectations the obstetrician must deal with the omnipresent threat of malpractice litigation. A less than perfect result often results in a lawsuit. The threat is real. The growth of malpractice suits is staggering. In 1970 in California there were five jury awards in excess of $300,000. The first malpractice award to exceed one million dollars in that state occurred in 1967. There have been more than 100 such awards since that time. Nationwide in 1982 there were an estimated two billion dollars in malpractice claims.[4]

Of course, not all of these awards are the result of childbirth-related incidents. However, few malpractice suits carry larger awards than those involving brain damage to a fetus or newborn. Money damages in such cases are calculated on the basis of providing lifetime rehabilitation, therapy, and private care, and are often in the multi-million dollar range. Lawyers who are compensated by receiving a percentage of such awards (the contingent fee) are attracted to such suits and pursue them with zeal—sometimes with little regard for the merits of who, if anyone, is at fault.

These considerations ultimately translate into money concerns for the doctor. Annual malpractice premiums for an obstetrician typically amount to $25,000 in California. If the physician is actually sued, his premiums may increase substantially, even if he is not at fault. Malpractice insurance pays for the lawyer who defends the doctor, and that cost, in the long run, also affects the level of malpractice premiums.

There are other, less obvious, costs of litigation. The doctor will have to spend time away from his practice testifying at his deposition or responding to interrogatories from the plaintiff's lawyer. The doctor's reputation may be adversely affected as his patients and peers learn of his involvement in suit. His practice may shrink as wary patients go to competitors and colleagues become reluctant to make referrals. All of this can happen before the case ever reaches a jury. Often the doctor will even be denied the opportunity of vindication as the practicalities and risks of litigation will dictate an out-of-court settlement. If the case proceeds to trial, the doctor may have to sit through a lengthy court proceeding in order to avoid a perception by the jury of indifference on his part to the plight of the injured child or mother. Finally, not the least cost of litigation is the emotional distress, frustration and anger experienced by the doctor as he proceeds through a system seemingly designed for, and only understood by, the lawyers.

Dr. Sandberg states, with only partial exaggeration:

> "Through this impetus (litigation) practice habits change and new standards of patient care emerge, not by intent and not under the scrutinizing eye of any one charged with improving the quality of medical care, but unintentionally and unknowingly by an array of juries and courts."[5]

The implications of this to VBAC's becomes clear when it is understood that essentially all obstetricians recognize that physicians are almost never sued for erring in the direction of cesarean delivery.[6]

Of course, hospitals are generally named as defendants in malpractice suits along with the physicians. Consequently, hospital administrators can be expected to discourage the use of hospital facilities for VBAC's as long as the medical community perceives that this procedure carries a higher legal risk than do repeat cesareans.

There is no immediate solution to the burgeoning number of malpractice suits. To a large extent it is up to the legislatures and courts of the various states to take the situation in hand. Until a solution is found, the risk of litigation will continue to be a factor mitigating against VBAC's.

THE EMOTIONAL ASPECTS

In addition to legal, practical, and philosophical considerations in choosing the mode of birth, the emotional aspects must enter into the considerations. How you feel about delivering vaginally is important.

Many women are not interested in a trial of labor. They feel that if they prepare for a cesarean birth, exercising their options, and perhaps sharing the birth with the father or another special person, it can be a positive and fulfilling experience. For them the decision to have a scheduled repeat cesarean would be the right decision.

However, many other women feel strongly that they would prefer to deliver vaginally. Nancy Cohen, founder of C/SEC, INC., runs counseling classes for cesarean couples seeking a VBAC (she coined the term *VBAC*). Cohen, who has herself had two VBAC's, says,

> Individually or in classes I have counseled well over a hundred women. All but three of them had vaginal births. This country has an attitude that women aren't capable of giving birth without tools, tubes, and machines. Women are frightened, tense, and tight. I believe most cesareans can be prevented, and certainly most repeats aren't necessary. We work on attitude, pain confrontation, emotions, creating a positive environment, all with the aim of allowing a woman to relax. We stress nutrition, exercise, vitamins, and relaxation techniques. I believe there is an inseparable relationship between the mind and the body and that birth is just as spiritual as it is physical.[7]

Comments from some of Cohen's students show that many women feel very strongly about delivering vaginally even after a cesarean. "Having a cesarean," said Lois Estner, "was like being dressed for the prom and getting hit by a truck. I didn't finish what I set out to do. This time we would really like to experience a vaginal birth." Her husband Martin added, "Our friends and relatives were shocked. Why can't we do this like everybody else? It's heretical to downgrade medical procedures that most people are convinced are advantageous."[8] "Nobody should categorically decide on my fate," said Marilyn Silverman, "and tell me I have to have a repeat cesarean."[9]

What is the trial of labor really like? Certainly no two women will have the exact same experience, but the following are two true stories with different endings. One mother had a successful VBAC and the other relates a story of a trial of labor that ends in a cesarean delivery.

Barbara Kalmen,[10] who had two cesareans before a VBAC, tells us:

"My labor started one month early and it was discovered the baby was in a breech presentation. So my first baby was born by cesarean. My baby was taken from my body and whisked away. My arms were empty, my stomach sore, my husband not there. The birth had a hollow feeling to it. It was like a beautiful bell but with the clapper missing.

"When I first became pregnant again I knew that I did not want another cesarean. I wanted my family to be together, not taken apart and separated. I put an enormous amount of time and energy into planning that birth. My options for both a vaginal and a cesarean birth were clearly spelled out. After numerous, detailed meetings with the hospital administration, they finally approved having my husband present if I had a cesarean birth. Again labor began one month early. Twenty-four hours passed. During eighteen of those hours I had contractions three-four minutes apart. I felt frustrated that labor did not progress (I made it to three-four cm. and remained there for eight hours). I was disappointed that another cesarean was necessary, but resigned myself to creating a positive birth anyway. Paul and I were together. We held hands until our baby was born and then gazed upon her in awe. She did not leave our side until I was wheeled from the operating room, and then we were separated for only ten minutes. She nursed for more than an hour in the recovery room and we went home forty hours after her birth. Part of the empty feeling inside me began to fill.

"But I still felt the second birth was not the best or the most fulfilling experience a birth could be. Even when telling everyone how wonderful everything was at the birth I still felt like I'd missed something. I have taught dozens of people how to give birth vaginally, something I was unable to do myself. I had healthy children and almost felt guilty wanting more from a birth. I felt jealous of my friends who have given birth naturally. I felt less than female. Yes, I'd done the conceiving, the carrying, but the birth was done by others. I felt like an artist. I had mixed the colors, arranged them on the canvas, and then someone else had signed the painting.

"With this pregnancy I decided I would attempt a VBAC, but I was afraid the birth would be another cesarean and I would still feel empty, still not quite complete. My belly grew and grew. My due date came and went. Already this baby was different. I was actually 'overdue' and waiting. The telephone became an annoyance as friends checked up on me.

"If I had not been so committed to a VBAC, I might have already had this baby. I would have just scheduled my cesarean and been done with the waiting and the concern. I feared that I would wait all this time and a cesarean would still be necessary.

"The fear, although small, picked away at my confidence as each day passed. How could I justify another Cesarean to myself? Many of my friends had had successful VBAC's I worried about my body being big enough as the baby gained ounces each day. The female in me wanted to be confirmed to just do what millions of other women have done before. The pressure of this baby inside me was light as a feather compared to the weight on my mind and soul.

"Ten days after my due date I was getting out of a chair when my bag of waters broke. I was frightened, but there was no turning back. I was riding on a roller coaster that had a track to follow, and I was strapped in the seat. Paul arrived home from work shortly after; my contractions were now every four minutes. Paul's hands, his words, his encouragement were part of a healing that took place that night.

"The labor was fast and intense. I was surprised at how crystal clear I felt inside my head, like the dawn after a night rainstorm. My eyes were closed almost all of the time. I was flowing with an ocean inside me. Storms would come and last a minute or so, and then a calm would descend, leaving the water with ripples that matched my breathing. I felt like an experienced sailor who knows the power of the storm, but also knows how to handle the boat to stay on course.

"We gathered what we could and headed for the hospital, a fifteen minute drive. When we arrived, I was really pushing; the baby was pushing. It was hard to tell which or who was in control, but I knew then that I would have this baby vaginally.

"Another exam revealed what I already knew: I was completely dilated and my baby would be born soon. I felt my vaginal area being stretched so tight. When my doctor decided to do an episiotomy I no longer cared. I felt the pressure release as the baby slid forward. (No medication was given. Pressure episiotomy really works—there was no pain there.) I reached down and picked up this incredibly warm, squirming creature. A cough, and a small cry of protest, of greeting, was uttered by her as I laid her on my breast. Only forty minutes had passed since we had arrived in the labor room. Paul stood beside me beaming. Our energies had melded, I felt more one with Paul than I ever had before.

"I had finally done it! Nine pounds one ounce of healthy baby had channeled through me into this world, and I had given my best to make it a safe passage. The void that had been inside me for eight years was no more! Instead, a bubbling well of love for this little person was springing up inside me. I felt content. A feeling of completeness and accomplishment swelled within me like a flower in full bloom."

Women who have had a cesarean birth never take a vaginal birth for granted. For this reason often their senses are heightened and their appreciation of the experience more intense.

Many mothers will go through a trial of labor and it will still result in a cesarean birth. This is a disappointing experience, as related by one mother:

"I always knew I would try again to have a vaginal birth after my first baby was delivered by cesarean. When I became pregnant the second time I immediately began to prepare for a VBAC. I was motivated largely by my desire to experience a vaginal birth as we had already taken a natural childbirth class the first time I was pregnant, and also I was motivated by my conviction that I shouldn't just automatically have a repeat cesarean simply because my first was that way. My doctor had never done a VBAC and he was not willing to try one with me even though he agreed with me that I would be a good candidate.

"My husband and I worked so hard for this VBAC. We eventually found a good doctor who would allow a trial of labor. I had to travel many miles to see him and I had to travel 30 miles to go to a hospital that would take me. Distances were always a big worry to us.

"After all this effort and 18 hours of labor I had to have a cesarean again, and for the same reason as the first time (malposition).

"It has been four months since all this happened and I am still not over it yet. I know I will get over it in time. I have so much support from my husband, family, and friends. But the fact remains that a mother who wants a VBAC at this point in time usually has to fight so hard for it and she is subject to so much worry and stress, and then when labor ends up in another cesarean, well, it's very hard to take. You are just left with the feeling that there has to be a better way and the medical community isn't doing as much about it as they should be. So, I just have some residual anger and frustration left to work out. I do not want to discourage women from attempting a VBAC, but this side of the story should be heard."

These two stories give you something to consider. As an expectant couple you can look at these two views and consider your own situation. In many decisions there are risks to weigh against benefits, and against the risks of the alternatives. The evaluation process may consist of weighing a medical risk against a spiritual or psychological risk, or a risk to the mother against a risk to the baby, and so on. There often is not an obvious answer.

When planning any part of your birth experience you would be wise to consult with the appropriate professionals in the area of your option: the obstetrician, the anesthesiologist, the nutritionist, and the pediatrician. Share your ideas and feelings with them.

The doctor's input into the decision-making process will be based on his experience and medical knowledge. Your contribution to the decision will be based on your value system, the information you have, and your individual personality and needs. In most instances, we believe the final decision can be arrived at jointly.

Nancy Krauter, President of the New York Cesarean Birth Association, sums it up when she says,

"We encourage couples to do their research, talk to their doctors, know their options, recognize their emotional biases, then make educated decisions. Either way, they should make sure the doctor and the hospital they have chosen offer the features they want. For example, for a repeat perhaps they want a family-centered hospital. For a trial labor, they should have a clear understanding with the doctor as to how he is going to measure progress in labor and at what point he plans to intervene."[11]

VBAC PARENTS' SPECIAL NEEDS— WHAT TO EXPECT

Parents deciding that they want to try a VBAC need special consideration. On an emotional level they need to understand and ACCEPT that a trial of labor may possibly result in another cesarean birth. Think for a moment. If you have gone through all the preparation for a natural childbirth, and then you go through the labor process, with the pain and the nervousness that would be associated with the VBAC, and all this ends up in a surgical birth after all—you know this will be traumatic.

As cesarean parents who desire a vaginal birth, you may harbor many negative feelings resulting from the past cesarean. You need the opportunity to make known your concerns and expectations for the upcoming birth.

Routine labor and delivery procedures should be discussed. The use of oxytocin augmentation and epidural anesthesia with internal toco-dynamic and internal monitoring should be explained to you by your doctor or childbirth instructor. A childbirth instructor would also be invaluable in teaching you breathing and relaxation techniques to help you through your trial of labor.

Finally, it is vital for the mother to enter the hospital when contractions are regular and of increasing intensity. You definitely do not want to risk a home birth. If you have never experienced labor before you should have your doctor describe labor signs. If you are in doubt, go to the hospital. Remember, if you have any vaginal bleeding, or your "bag of waters" breaks, you should immediately depart for the hospital.

Intrapartal Period

Upon entering the hospital, you will be immediately placed on external fetal monitoring to check uterine contractions and fetal well-being. An intravenous will be started in the event that you should require fluids, blood, or medication quickly.

The anesthesia and nursery personnel are alerted that you have arrived and a trial of labor has begun. You must be adequately informed of the trial of labor process and its risks, and must give your consent. Two units of blood must be available, and finally, the attending physician and hospital staff must be prepared to perform a cesarean, should it become necessary, within 15 to 20 minutes. Since surgery and a general anesthesia may be necessary, you will be asked to limit oral intake to small amounts of ice chips. An antacid may be given every 3 or 4 hours to neutralize stomach acidity.

When your bag of waters breaks, you will be given a vaginal exam. Then, in order to assess fetal well-being and the strength of your contractions, a fetal scalp electrode and an intrauterine pressure catheter are inserted into the uterus. A nurse will watch these constantly to see how you and the baby are doing. These are more senstive than the external monitors and permit the nurse to accurately ascertain the pressure on your uterine scar. Abdominal pain alone is an unreliable indicator of uterine rupture because the pain can be due to too many difficult things. Also, some women do not experience pain with uterine ruptures.

At this point in time only minimal amounts of analgesics are administered to the mother during the trial of labor to avoid masking the pain of uterine rupture. Epidural anesthesia is usually avoided for the same reason. However, as just mentioned, pain is not a reliable indicator of uterine rupture and the results of a new study indicate that it is perhaps safer to use analgesics than previously thought.[11]

Maternal vital signs should be monitored once or twice every half hour, and temperature every two hours. To deal with pain, you will be encouraged to use breathing and relaxation techniques. Other procedures to relieve discomfort include back rubs, cold cloths administered to your brow and some help in getting into comfortable positions until the birth is imminent.

As in any delivery, failure for labor to progress, or fetal distress may cause labor to be terminated and a cesarean performed.

After the vaginal birth the uterine scar must be evaluated by the doctor. He will make an internal exam to check the old scar and make sure it is intact.

Postpartum Care

After the delivery you will be moved to the recovery room and observed very closely to make sure you do not have an undetected uterine rupture which would result in heavy vaginal bleeding. At least every fifteen minutes for the first hour following delivery your vital signs, fundal status (firmness) and a description of vaginal discharge will be recorded and evaluated. Any abnormality in the above could indicate that you experienced some degree of uterine rupture, and your doctor will be immediately notified.

If you remain stable in the recovery room, then your care would be the same as for any woman having a vaginal delivery.

VBAC—THE FUTURE

The increasing cesarean rate has been of mounting public concern. Nonetheless, except for a handful of doctors and health care professionals, the medical profession has ignored or disregarded the recent studies that indicate that VBAC's are safer under many circumstances. The continually escalating cesarean birth rate is evidence of this fact.

Some doctors have expressed alarm at the lack of acceptance by their peers of VBAC's. A December, 1984, article in the *Journal of the American Medical Association* reported on the recommendation of a consensus development conference of the National Institutes of Health in 1980. The recommendations were expected to lead to a decrease in the cesarean birthrate. The *Journal* said:

> "Prior cesarean delivery, recognized as the second most frequent cause for cesarean birth, has recently been the subject of discussion. The consensus development conference clearly stated:
>
> 'In hospitals with appropriate facilities, services and staff for prompt emergency cesarean birth, a proper selection of cases should permit a safe trial of labor and vaginal delivery for women who have had a previous low segment transverse cesarean birth. . . .'
>
> It may be expected that such a statement should lead to a change in practice patterns throughout the country. This does not seem, however, to have occurred. The rule in the majority of hospitals is still 'once a cesarean section, always a cesarean section.' It is important to note that the consensus development conference also stated:
>
> 'In hospitals without the proper facilities, services and staff, the risk of a trial of labor in a woman who has had a previous cesarean may exceed the risk for both mother and infant from a properly timed, elective repeat cesarean birth. Patients should be informed in advance of the limits of a particular institution's capabilities and of the availability of other institutions capable of offering this service so that they may make a choice.'
>
> With repeated cesarean section rates still running at or close to 100% in many institutions, undoubtedly neither of these recommendations has achieved wide acceptance."[12]

Despite the overwhelming evidence that VBAC's are safe in many circumstances, and despite the fact that a VBAC is in the best interest of many expectant mothers, a trial of labor simply is not an option for most women. Women have to struggle for the opportunity to try a VBAC.

The facts are in! VBAC is as safe, indeed safer, for many women as a cesarean delivery. Armed with the recent guidelines issued by the American College of Obstetrics and Gynecology, prospective parents should be instrumental in reversing the escalating upward trend of cesarean births. The medical profession will respond to consumer pressure for change. If not, the *Journal* article may prove to be profoundly prophetic:

> "Unless the medical community initiates a review process of cesarean section rates, others will press for outside review. The medical community should establish a mechanism that will result in acceptable cesarean section rates before legislation does."[13]

CHAPTER SEVENTEEN

Getting It Your Way

This book is intended to be a guide to achieving a fulfilling, enriching, and happy birth experience. We have discussed various birth options and choices and provided you with information to help you make decisions based on the facts available at this time. This final chapter is designed to act as a guide in choosing your doctors and hospital. It also contains suggestions on how to approach your doctor on the subject of a father-attended cesarean birth (FACB) and/or a vaginal birth after a cesarean (VBAC).

GETTING AN FACB

If you are fortunate enough to be in an area where FACB is available, your sole job will be to choose among the various doctors and hospitals that allow this procedure. However, this is an important job and will take some investigation. For this reason, you should begin early in your pregnancy. You may already have an obstetrician, but just because he delivered your last baby or a friend recommended him or he is located nearby does not necessarily mean that he would be the best choice for your FACB. You may have to interview a variety of doctors before finding one you feel is a qualified surgeon and who shares your philosophy about shared birth.

Fortunately, more and more doctors are welcoming parent participation. The attitude of many doctors was well put by the chief of obstetrics at a major university medical center recently:

I believe that parents should have all the information on cesarean birth they possibly can have, such as complications and possible risks, so if or when it gets down to a decision on the course of management they can participate in a meaningful way. Many times there is not an "always right" answer to a problem. There are choices to be made. Most choices involve risks of different sorts. Doctors have to weigh one risk against another. The parents being involved in these decisions can help a lot. It becomes a shared responsibility, and that's good when you sometimes have to make a big decision based on a small bit of information.[1]

When you find a doctor who shares these sentiments you have the basis for a good working relationship.

Some suggestions for selecting an obstetrician (OB) include obtaining recommendations from your local cesarean support group or from another doctor whom you trust, perhaps your family doctor. After you make your list, check on the credentials of the doctors you have preliminarily selected. Find out where they went to medical school and did their residencies. Make sure they are diplomates (not just fellows) of the American Board of Obstetrics and Gynecology.

Once you have satisfied yourself of the professional qualifications of your list of candidates, it is time to begin making appointments to talk to them. If your husband is going to accompany you, let the doctor's office know at the time you set up the appointment. It is advisable that your husband visit with the doctor *at least once* during your pregnancy. The doctor may not charge you for this initial interview, but some doctors do.

To get the maximum benefit from your interview you should know before your visit what you want to communicate to the doctor. Before the visit, you and your husband should discuss what you feel your ideal birth experience would be like. Make a list of your requests. Decide together which requests are most important to you and on which ones you would be willing to compromise. Explain your requests to the doctor. For example, you might say, "I would like very much to spend the night before surgery at home with my family. I would appreciate it if this could be arranged with the hospital." You can go on to explain your reasons. It is important to select a doctor with whom you and your husband can talk comfortably.

You should select your pediatrician with the same care you select your OB. Discuss your requests with him (or her), too. He is the one who is medically responsible for the baby from the moment it is born. Ask him about his routine procedures and policies for cesarean babies.

If you have a choice of hospitals for your FACB, find out what options they provide cesarean families. Some options you might consider are:

1. Doing a partial prep

2. Arranging an opportunity to talk with the anesthesiologist before surgery

3. Allowing the father to attend the birth (FACB)

4. Permitting the father to stand up and watch the birth of the baby

5. Allowing the mother to be awake for the birth of the baby

6. Letting the mother witness the birth of the baby via a mirror

7. Allowing photographs to be taken

8. Allowing the mother to see, hold, and/or nurse the baby in the operating room

9. Performing initial baby care within mother's view

10. Having the option of a Leboyer bath*

11. Inviting the father to watch the initial care of baby while the pediatrician explains what he is doing

12. Giving the baby to the father to hold and bring to his wife to see

13. Allowing the father to visit the mother and baby in the recovery room, or the baby in the nursery

14. Letting the father visit at any time during waking hours

15. "Rooming-in" (the baby stays in the mother's room) with help in caring for the baby from the father, nurse, or surrogate

16. Permitting your other children to visit you in the hospital

Finally, when you choose a hospital, consider costs. They do vary from one hospital to another.

---

*Leboyer is a French doctor who believes that the birth experience is traumatic to the newborn and that consequently the baby may develop problems later in life. He developed a special method of delivery in an effort to lessen the effects of the transition from the mother's womb to the environment of the delivery room. Leboyer's recommendations include: a warm and quiet delivery room, dimmed lighting, gentle handling of the newborn, immediate positioning of the baby on the mother's abdomen (cesarean mothers will have to devise another method of skin to skin contact; fathers may fill in for this), delay in cutting the umbilical cord until the pulsation has stopped, and placing the newborn in a warm tub of water. All these measures are taken in an effort to duplicate the environment in the mother's womb and make the birth transition smoother and less painful for the infant.

After your hospital has been selected, make sure that you and your husband get a tour of the operating room before surgery. Maternity teas for cesarean couples and childbirth classes routinely provide this, but if you do not get the opportunity through these channels, contact the head nurse at the hospital and ask her to arrange a tour for you.

WHAT TO DO IF FACB IS NOT PRACTICED IN YOUR AREA

If you want a FACB, but after researching your community you find it has not previously been available, do not despair. Getting FACB started in your area can initially be somewhat frustrating and time consuming but can also be an exciting and fulfilling project, as many "pioneer couples" can tell you. If you feel strongly about the FACB concept you may want to see it started in your area. A good initial step is to send to the Cesarean Birth Council, International, for its information package. Write to Cesarean Birth Council, International, P.O. Box 4331, Mountain View, California 94040. Among other things, this package contains convincing letters from an obstetrician, an anesthesiologist, and a pediatrician on the benefits of FACB.

Armed with this literature, visit the doctors you have selected. The manner in which you approach your doctor can make a big difference in how receptive he (or she) will be to your ideas. It is not a good idea to seek a confrontation. If you present your views defiantly, he will be happy to see you go elsewhere regardless of his personal philosophy about having babies might be.

You will be more convincing if you and your husband go to the doctor together and make your request in a confident, dignified, and friendly way. If you are having a repeat cesarean, you might say, "We are aware that in some instances fathers have been allowed in the surgical suite with their wives to lend support and to witness the birth of their baby. We would like this kind of birth experience for ourselves. How do you suggest we proceed toward that goal?" A doctor is much more likely to be receptive to this approach than to the mother appearing alone, saying apologetically, "Can my husband be with me in surgery?" or angrily demanding your husband's presence in the operating room.

If you are planning for natural childbirth but want to be sure your husband can be with you in the event of an emergency cesarean, you will want to approach the obstetrician in a similar fashion: "My husband and I are preparing for a father-attended cesarean birth as well as for a vaginal birth. In the event I would have to have a cesarean, under what circumstances would you permit us to share this birth experience? These are some of our requests."

Now you have introduced the idea. Maybe you will have to give the doctor some time to think it over. In the meantime, ask other interested parents and professionals to write letters or discuss the subject with him and the hospital administrator.

If you feel your doctor doesn't respect your view, write for *The Final Report of the Consensus Development Task Force on Cesarean Childbirth*. This report is available free by writing to Ms. Pam Driscoll, Office of Research Reporting, Bldg. 31, Room 2A 32, National Institute of Health, Rockville Pike, Bethesda, Maryland 20205.

This report comes from the National Institute of Health which formed a development task force on cesarean childbirth. This task force was made up of experts from relevant fields, of which there were six obstetricians, twelve physicians, a member of C/SEC's professional advisory board, one lawyer, and one consumer parent. These experts met periodically last year to address the following questions: (1) How and why have cesarean delivery rates changed in the United States and elsewhere? (2) What is the evidence that a cesarean delivery improves the outcome of various complications of pregnancy? (3) What are the medical and psychological effects of cesarean delivery on the mother, infant, and family? (4) What economic factors are related to the rising cesarean rate? and (5) What legal and ethical considerations are involved in decisions on cesarean delivery?

The following is a partial list of the recommendations.

1. Parent education during pregnancy by health care providers and in childbirth education classes should include information relating to the possibility of a cesarean birth, an explanation of the technical procedures surrounding the cesarean birth, and discussion of choices available to parents.

2. During labor and at the time a decision to perform a cesarean is made, as time and circumstances permit, a discussion of the indications, procedures, and parental options should take place between the physician or his or her staff and the parents.

3. Information exchange about the entire cesarean birth experience should continue in the postoperative period and at later postpartum visits.

4. In the absence of scientific evidence regarding benefit or risk, the presence at a cesarean birth of the father or surrogate should represent a joint decision among parents, physician, and hospital representatives.

5. Hospitals are encouraged to liberalize their policies concerning the option of having the father or surrogate attend the cesarean birth.

6. The healthy neonate should not be separated routinely from mother and father following delivery.[2]

You can also consider starting a cesarean support group. A group is often more effective than an individual in changing policies and attitudes. If you want to form a cesarean group, write to C/SEC, Inc., 66 Christopher Road, Waltham, Massachusetts 02154 for the *Guide for Establishing and Running a Support Group.*

And you can contact the local childbirth instructors and ask that a class on FACB be made a part of the curriculum in prepared childbirth classes. This extra class would prepare repeat cesarean couples as well as those couples who expect vaginal birth but who end up having a cesarean. C/SEC, Inc., has a manual entitled *Setting Up Prepared Childbirth Classes for Cesarean Parents.*

Trainex Corporation has an excellent film documentary, entitled ''Make Room for Dad,'' on the father-attended cesarean birth available in the format of your choice. You can write to Trainex Corporation, P.O. Box 116, Garden Grove, California 92642, or call California toll-free (800) 472-2479 or national toll-free (800) 854-2485.

With these efforts, you can probably convince a well-qualified doctor to allow you to have a shared cesarean birth even if it is not currently being practiced in your area. The doctor may choose to quietly allow your husband to be with you in the operating room before there is any official change in hospital policy. This is the way it starts in many instances. Then, as the benefits of FACB become evident, an adjustment in attitudes evolves and FACB becomes the official policy of the hospital.

PLANNING FOR A VBAC

Basically the same principles apply in arranging for a VBAC that you would employ in arranging for a FACB, such as the need to be informed, persistent, and committed to your goal, and to approach your doctor in an open and tactful manner.

There are, however, some significant differences. For a safe VBAC the hospital *must* have certain facilities. There must be 24-hour, in-house coverage by blood bank personnel. Anesthesiologists or anesthetists and operating personnel must be able to do a cesarean delivery within 30 minutes once it is indicated. If your hospital cannot meet these qualifications, perhaps you should change hospitals anyway. Dr. Klein of the American College of Obstetrics and Gynecology has been quoted as saying, "trial of labor requires sustained services that keep other laboring patients and their infants safe. Emergencies arising from hemorrhage, prolapsed cord, or fetal distress will occur wherever babies are delivered and will occur more frequently than symptomatic rupture of the uterus in patients properly selected for a trial of labor." Teaching hospitals with residents in obstetrics and anesthesiology on duty at all times, day and night, are the most likely settings for a VBAC. In many hospitals, the staff mentioned are usually "on call" and live within ten to fifteen minutes of the hospital.

Perhaps before you spend a lot of time searching for the right hospital you should make sure you are a candidate for a VBAC. To do this, you will have to get complete records from your previous delivery. Your doctor will look at these records to determine the kind of incision you have on your uterus. You need to have a low cervical transverse incision. The doctor needs to know if you had any operative or postoperative complications such as fever or infection. And, last of all, he needs to know the reason for your past cesarean (see Chapter 16 on VBAC for more information about this). Your previous cesarean must have been necessitated by a condition for which a repeat cesarean is not mandated, such as breech presentations, fetal distress, or toxemia.

Assuming you are a candidate for a VBAC and you have found a hospital, the next thing to do is to find the right doctor. Hopefully, your present doctor will be willing to try a VBAC. However, there is a good chance he does not deliver babies at a hospital that is equipped and/or willing to do VBAC's. If that is the case, you will have to change doctors. Hospitals that permit VBAC's can supply you with a list of obstetricians on their staffs. You might ask the maternity supervisor to indicate which ones are likely to favor a VBAC. Sometimes it is hard to change from a doctor whom you know and trust to a less familiar one. You might be able to arrange for your former doctor to consult with your new doctor, thus easing the transition. Be forewarned. Changing doctors can get expensive, because you may have to interview many before you find the right one for your VBAC.

Finding the Right Doctor

The doctor you are looking for should sympathize with your desire to have a VBAC. He should be medically qualified, and ideally he or she will have some experience with VBAC. Because VBAC's are not commonly done in this country, most doctors have no firsthand experience. Their experience may be limited to what they have read in medical journals or heard at medical conferences.

When you find a doctor who says he will attempt a VBAC, you might consider asking him some of the following questions to determine the level of his commitment. "How long will I be allowed to labor?" "What sort of things would lead you to decide that the trial of labor be terminated and a cesarean be performed?" and "When would you start timing my labor?" These are difficult questions for a doctor to answer absolutely. Don't expect pat answers. Many variables affect his decision, and each situation has to be judged individually.

After reviewing some of the problems associated with "getting it your way" in regard to VBAC, you are probably asking yourself some hard questions about how much it means to you to attempt it at all. There is yet one more question to answer: "Am I willing to experience unmedicated labor?" You will not be medicated because it it important for you to be able to feel discomfort or pain between contractions, which are symptoms of uterine rupture.

As we researched the problem, we concluded that unless things fell in place extremely well, it might take more than your nine months of pregnancy to arrange for a VBAC. It would be a good idea to start planning for a VBAC before you become pregnant so you may be cared for by the same doctor during your entire pregnancy if you should have to change from your present doctor. Also, then you can relax during your entire pregnancy without unnecessary stress and leg work to tax your energy.

One last word of advice. If you are planning a VBAC, also plan for the possibility of a cesarean, including an FACB, anesthesia preference, and so on, and have your doctor include your options and preferences on your chart. Your overall goal in planning your birth should be to have the best possible, be it vaginal or cesarean. Trust your doctor and approach your birth with joy.

Finally, we urge you not to hold rigid expectations about this approaching delivery, be it a FACB or VBAC. Anything can change at any time, and rigid expectations only make it difficult for you to adjust.

AFTER THE BIRTH

You worked and planned for the birth of your baby, an event that has special meaning to you. If you were unhappy over the birth due to ill treatment on the part of the doctors, nurses, or hospital, write a letter and tell them so. Join the local cesarean group. You may have to start one in your community. Work with them to bring about changes in hospital policies regarding cesarean birth and to increase the awareness of the health professionals to the special needs and concerns of cesarean parents.

If you are happy with your experience, and the chances are you will be as a result of your effort, interest, and care in working with your doctor and hospital in preparation for this occasion, don't forget to also write to your doctor, birth instructor, and hospital and let them know that you appreciate their concern and their enlightened approach to cesarean care. Praise is far more powerful than criticism in effecting change. Your positive feedback may give them the necessary encouragement to change some other aspects of patient care in favor of the consumer. This book began with some letters from dissatisfied consumers, to which many of you could relate. Now we would like to share this letter with you:

January 30, 1978

Mr. James Deutsch
Westlake Community Hospital
4415 Lakeview Canyon Road
Westlake Village, California 91361

Dear Mr. Deutsch:

I am writing this letter on behalf of my wife and myself to express our sincere and grateful appreciation for the care and treatment of my wife and new baby daughter during their recent stay at your hospital. The personal attention that they received was outstanding. The warm atmosphere generated by the nurses was a definite aid in my wife's recuperation from a cesarean.

I would like to take this opportunity to thank you for your policy which allows the husband to participate in a cesarean birth. It was an experience that I will treasure for the rest of my life. The physicians were extremely thoughtful and considerate during the surgery. They made me feel that I was really a part of my daughter's birth instead of an unwanted third party. I cannot begin to express how I felt when the doctor handed me my daughter only minutes after her birth.

The cesarean childbirth classes at your hospital were most helpful in preparing Leslie and myself for the surgery. Knowing what was going to happen made the experience one of happiness and joy instead of fear and anxiety.

Very sincerely yours,

Harry Leff

Across the country, concerned couples have banded together to change the traditional approach to cesarean birth. Through their efforts, cesarean childbirth can now become a family experience. A more humanistic and fulfilling cesarean experience can be achieved. With some careful thought, education, planning, and determination you, too, can achieve a joyful birth experience. We wish each one of you a very happy and special "birth" day!

Notes

Chapter 2

1. The American College of Obstetrics and Gynecology new guidelines for VBAC.

2. William Hindle, "Round Table Discussion: Cesarean Section," *American Journal of Obstetrics and Gynecology*, Vol 149 (May 1, 1984), p. 42.

3. David N. Danforth, ed., *Obstetrics and Gynecology*, 3rd ed. (New York: Harper & Row, 1977), p. 12.

4. Danforth, p. 12.

5. J. Willson, C. Beecham, and E. Carrington, *Obstetrics and Gynecology* (St. Louis: Mosby, 1966), p. 557.

6. Danforth, p. 12.

7. Danforth, pp. 13–14.

8. Willson, Beecham, and Carrington, p. 557.

9. Bonnie Donovan, *The Cesarean Birth Experience* (Boston: Beacon Press, 1978).

10. Association for Family-Centered Cesareans, Authors' files.

11. Linda Prendergast and Suzanne Rosno, *Cesarean Beginnings: A Handbook for Parents and Professionals* (Saratoga, Calif.: Beginnings Publications, 1979), p. 15.

Chapter 3

1. Tracy Hotchner, *Pregnancy and Childbirth* (New York: Avon, 1979), p. 72.

2. This section is adapted from California Department of Health, *Nutrition During Pregnancy and Lactation* (Sacramento: California Department of Health, 1977), pp. 37–41.

3. *Recipe for Healthy Babies*, March of Dimes Birth Defects Foundation, 1275 Mamaroneck Ave., White Plains, NY 10605. No date.

4. California Department of Health, p. 90.

5. Hotchner, p. 76.

6. Cherilyn Sheets, personal communication, September 20, 1980.

7. J. Willis, "Misused Antibiotic Nothing to Smile About," *FDA Consumer,* March 1980, pp. 8–9.

Chapter 4

1. California Department of Health, *Nutrition During Pregnancy and Lactation* (Sacramento: California Department of Health, 1977), p. 19.

2. M. Shearer, "Malnutrition in Middle-Class Pregnant Women," *Birth and the Family Journal,* 1980, 7:27.

3. Shearer, pp. 33–34.

Chapter 5

1. Elizabeth Bing, *Moving Through Pregnancy* (New York: Bantam Books, 1976).

Chapter 6

1. D. Affonso, "Cesarean Birth: Women's Reactions," *American Journal of Nursing,* March 1980, p. 469.

2. J. Marut, "Comparison of Primiparas' Perceptions of Vaginal and Cesarean Births," *Nursing Research,* 1979, *28:264.*

3. Marut, p. 265.

4. Authors' files.

5. Affonso, p. 469.

6. This section relies heavily on M. McCaffery, *Nursing Management of the Patient with Pain* (Philadelphia: Lippincott, 1972), pp. 170–176.

7. Fitzhugh Dodson, *How to Parent* (New York: Signet, 1970), p. 129.

8. Haim Ginott, *Between Parent and Child* (New York: Avon, 1969), p. 149.

9. M. Trause, "Birth in the Hospital: the Effect on the Sibling," *Birth and the Family Journal,* 1978, *5:207–210.*

10. L. Salk, *Preparing for Parenthood* (New York: Bantam Books, 1974), p. 50.

Chapter 7

1. Danforth, p. 495.

2. Danforth, p. 496.

3. National Institute of Child Health and Human Resource Development, National Institutes of Health, *Consensus Development Conference on*

Cesarean Childbirth: Draft Report of the Task Force on Cesarean Birth (Bethesda, Md.: National Institute of Child Health and Human Resource Development, National Institutes of Health, 1980), pp. 303–304.

4. F. Trigoletto, "Avoiding Iatrogenic Prematurity with Elective Repeat Cesarean Section Without the Routine Use of Amniocentesis," *American Journal of Obstetrics and Gynecology,* 1980, *137*:521–524.

5. Trigoletto, p. 524.

Chapter 8

1. National Institutes of Health, Public Health Service, U.S. Department of Health, Education and Welfare, *NIH Consensus Development Statement on Cesarean Childbirth* (Bethesda, Md.: National Institutes of Health, Public Health Service, 1980), p. 10.

2. National Institutes of Health, p. 12.

Chapter 10

1. Susan Sheridan, personal communication, September 1980.

Chapter 13

1. La Leche League International, *The Womanly Art of Breast feeding* (Franklin Park, Ill.: La Leche League International, 1976).

2. Karen Pryor, *Nursing Your Baby* (New York: Pocket Books, 1976).

3. Maternal and Child Health Branch, California Department of Health, *Policy Statement: Breastfeeding—Its Role in Infant Growth and Development* (Sacramento, Calif.: Maternal and Child Health Branch, California Department of Health, 1977), p. 1.

4. Pryor, pp. 29–30.

5. Pryor, p. 32.

6. La Leche League, p. 29.

7. Pryor, p. 155.

8. Pryor, p. 156.

9. Authors' files.

Chapter 14

1. Fitzhugh Dodson, *How to Parent* (New York: Signet, 1970), pp. 131–132.

2. Authors' files.

3. Tracy Hotchner, *Pregnancy and Childbirth* (New York: Avon, 1979), pp. 571–572.

Chapter 15

1. All material by Jack Klausen in this chapter was written especially for this book.

2. Authors' files.

3. Linda Prendergast and Suzanne Rosno, *Cesarean Beginnings: A Handbook for Parents and Professionals* (Saratoga, Calif.: Beginnings Publications, 1979), p. 16.

4. Prendergast and Rosno, p. 17.

5. All the following personal accounts in this chapter are from the authors' files.

Chapter 16

1. National Institute of Child Health and Human Resource Development, National Institute of Health, *Consensus Development Conference on Cesarean Childbirth: Draft Report of the Task Force on Cesarean Childbirth* (Bethesda, Md.: National Institute of Child Health and Human Development, National Institutes of Health, (1980), p. 343.

2. A. Richard Graham, "Trial of Labor Following Previous Cesarean Section," *American Journal of Obstetrics and Gynecology*, Vol 149 (May 1984), p. 36.

3. Bruce L. Flamm, "Use of Oxytocin Augmentation and Epidural Anesthesia with Internal Tocodynamics and Internal Fetal Monitoring," *The American Journal of Obstetrics and Gynecology*, Vol 148 (March 15, 1984), p. 763.

4. A. Richard Graham, "Trial of Labor Following Previous Cesarean Section," *American Journal of Obstetrics and Gynecology*, Vol 149 (May 1984), pg. 42.

5. Ibid.

6. Ibid.

7. J. Rattner Heilman, "Breaking the Cesarean Cycle," *New York Times Magazine*, (Sept. 7, 1980), p. 92.

8. Heilman, p. 92.

9. Heilman, p. 93.

10. Barbara Kalmen is a R.N., childbirth educator, co-founder and current president of C.A.R.E.S.S. (Cesarean Association for Research, Education, Support, and Satisfaction).

11. Bruce L. Flamm, "Use of Oxytocin Augmentation and Epidural Anesthesia with Internal Tocodynamics and Internal Fetal Monitor-

ing," *American Journal of Obstetrics and Gynecology*, Vol. 148 (March 15, 1984), p. 764.

12. Norbert Gleicher, "Cesarean Section Rates in the United States," *Journal of the American Medical Association*, Vol. 252 (Dec. 21, 1984), p. 3274.

13. Ibid., p. 3276.

Chapter 17

1. Authors' files.

2. National Institutes of Health, Public Health Service, U.S. Department of Health, Education and Welfare, *NIH Consensus Development Statement on Cesarean Childbirth*, (Bethesda, Md.: National Institutes of Health, Public Health Service, U.S. Department of Health, Education and Welfare, 1980), p. 18.

3. Luella Klein, "Cesarean Birth and Trial of Labor," *The Female Patient*, Vol. 9 (Sept. 1984), p. 117.

Appendix

1. Luis R. Saldana, Harold Schulman, and Lynn Reuss, "Management of Pregnancy After Cesarean Section," *American Journal of Obstetrics and Gynecology*, 1979, *135*(5):561.

2. Berkeley S. Merrill and C. E. Gibbs, "Planned Vaginal Delivery Following Cesarean Section," *Obstetrics and Gynecology*, 1978, *52*(1): 52.

3. Merrill and Gibbs, p. 52.

4. Merrill and Gibbs, p. 52.

Recommended Reading

Cesarean Childbirth

C/SEC Incorporated. *Frankly Speakly: A Pamphlet for Cesarean Couples.*

Donovan, Bonnie. *The Cesarean Birth Experience.* 1977.

Hausknecht, Richard, M.D., and Heilman, Joan. *Having a Cesarean Baby.* 1978.

Meyer, Linda. *The Cesarean (R)evolution.* 1979.

Prendergast, Linda, and Rosno, Suzanne. *Cesarean Beginnings.* 1979.

Wilson, Christine, and Hovey, Wendy. *Cesarean Childbirth.* 1980.

Breastfeeding

Applebaum, Richard. *Abreast of the Times.* 1970.

Brewster, Dorothy. *You Can Breastfeed Your Baby.* 1979.

Eiger, Marvin, and Olds, Sally. *The Complete Book of Breastfeeding.* 1972.

Ewy, Donna, and Ewy, Rodger. *Preparation for Breastfeeding,* 1975.

Kippley, Sheila. *Breastfeeding and Natural Child Spacing.* 1974.

La Leche League International. *The Womanly Art of Breastfeeding.* 1963.

Pryor, Karen. *Nursing Your Baby.* 1976.

Raphael, Dana. *The Tender Gift: Breastfeeding.* 1978.

Rice, Ilene. *Heartstart.* 1978.

Bonding

Klaus, Marshall, and Kennell, John. *Maternal-Infant Bonding.* 1978.

Montagu, Ashley. *Touching.* 1971.

Young, Diony. *Bonding: How Parents Become Attached to Their Baby*. 1978.

Nutrition

Davis, Adelle. *Let's Have Healthy Children*. 1951.

Goldbeck, Nikki. *As You Eat, So Your Baby Grows*. 1977.

Goldbeck, Nikki, and Goldbeck, David. *Supermarket Handbook*. 1973.

Goldbeck, Nikki, and Goldbeck, David. *The Dieter's Companion*. 1976.

Johnson, Roberta. *Mother's in the Kitchen*. 1971.

Kenda, Margaret, and Williams, Phyllis. *The Natural Baby Food Cook Book*. 1972.

Landsky, Vicki. *The Taming of the C.A.N.D.Y. Monster*. 1978.

Lappé, Frances. *Diet for a Small Planet*. 1975.

Long, James. *The Essential Guide to Prescription Drugs*. 1977.

Sforza-Brewer, Gail. *What Every Pregnant Woman Should Know: The Truth About Diet and Drugs in Pregnancy*. 1977.

Williams, Phyllis. *Nourishing Your Unborn Child*. 1974.

Worthington, Bonnie. *Nutrition in Pregnancy and Lactation*. 1977.

Exercise and Relaxation Techniques

Benson, Herbert. *The Relaxation Response*. 1976.

Bing, Elizabeth. *Moving Through Pregnancy*. 1975.

Dilfer, Carol. *Your Baby, Your Body*. 1977.

Jacobson, Edmund. *How to Relax and Have Your Baby*. 1959.

Noble, Elizabeth. *Essential Exercises for the Childbearing Year*. 1976.

Shandler, Nina, and Shandler, Michael. *Yoga for Pregnancy and Birth*. 1979.

How to Get What You Want

Belsky, Marvin. *How to Choose and Use Your Doctor*. 1979.

Billingsley, T. *How to Talk Back to Your Obstetrician*. 1978.

Boston Women's Health Book Collective. *Our Bodies, Ourselves*. 1976.

Breslow, Lori. *How to Get the Best Health Care for Your Money*. 1979.

Elkins, V. *Rights of the Pregnant Parent*. 1976.

Walton, V. E. *Have It Your Way*. 1978.

Pregnancy

Annis, Linda. *The Child Before Birth*. 1978.

Bing, Elizabeth. *Making Love During Pregnancy*. 1977.

Bittman, Sam, and Zalk, Sue. *Expectant Fathers*. 1980.

British Museum Staff. *Life Before Birth*. 1979.

Colman, Arthur, and Colman, Libby. *Pregnancy*. 1971.

Flanagan, Geraldine. *The First Nine Months of Life*. 1964.

Gots, Ronald, and Gots, Barbara. *Caring for Your Unborn Child*. 1977.

Hotchner, Tracy. *Pregnancy and Childbirth*. 1979.

Kahan, Stuart. *The Expectant Father's Survival Kit*. 1978.

Maternity Center Association. *A Baby Is Born*. 1964.

Montagu, Ashley. *Life Before Birth*. 1977.

Nilsson, Ingelman-Sundberg, and Nillson, Wirsen. *A Child Is Born*. 1966.

Robe, Lucy Barry. *Just So It's Healthy*. 1977.

Sasmor, Jeanette. *What Every Husband Should Know About Having a Baby*. 1972.

Smith, David. *Mothering Your Unborn Baby*. 1979.

Thompson, Carol. *Childbirth Today: Prepared and Positive*. 1978.

Wachstein, Alison. *Pregnant Moments*. 1979.

Child Care and Development

Arena, Jay, and Bachar, Miriam. *Child Safety Is No Accident*. 1978.

Barber, Virginia, and Skaggs, Merrill. *The Mother Person*. 1975.

Bessell, Harold, and Kelly, Thomas. *The Parent Book*. 1978.

Brazelton, T. Barry. *Infants and Mothers*. 1969.

Brazelton, T. Barry. *Toddlers and Parents*. 1974.

Brazelton, T. Barry. *Doctor and Child*. 1976.

Bricklin, Alice. *Mother Love*. 1976.

Briggs, Dorothy. *Your Child's Self Esteem*. 1975.

Burck, Francis. *Babysense*. 1979.

Caplan, Frank. *The First Twelve Months of Life*. 1973.

Caplan, Frank. *The Second Twelve Months of Life*. 1977.

Clarke, Jean. *Self-Esteem: A Family Affair*. 1978.

Consumers Guide editors. *The Complete Baby Book: A Total Guide to Buying Products, Toys, and Medical Services.* 1979.

Crary, Elizabeth. *Without Spanking or Spoiling.* 1979.

Dodson, Fitzhugh. *How to Parent.* 1970.

Dodson, Fitzhugh. *How to Father.* 1974.

Dodson, Fitzhugh. *How to Discipline—With Love.* 1977.

Fraiberg, Selma. *Every Child's Birthright.* 1977.

Fraiberg, Selma. *The Magic Years.* 1959.

Gordon, Ira. *Baby Learning Through Baby Play.* 1970.

Gordon, Ira. *Child Learning Through Child Play.* 1972.

Gordon, Ira. *Baby to Parent, Parent to Baby.* 1977.

Gordon, Thomas. *Parent Effectiveness Training.* 1970.

Gribbin, Trish. *Pajamas Don't Matter.* 1979.

Grobman, Joann. *Born to Love.* 1976.

Hagstrom, Julie, and Morrill, Joan. *Games Babies Play.* 1979.

Jackson, Jane, and Jackson, Joseph. *Infant Culture.* 1978.

Kelly, Marguerite, and Parsons, Elia. *The Mother's Almanac.* 1975.

Koch, Jaroslav. *Total Baby Development.* 1978.

Leach, Penelope. *Your Baby and Child.* 1978.

Leboyer, Frederick. *Loving Hands.* 1976.

Olness, Karen. *Raising Happy, Healthy Children.* 1977.

Smith, Helen. *Survival Handbook for Pre-School Mothers.* 1978.

White, Burton. *The First Three Years of Life.* 1975.

Appendix

ABSTRACT: MANAGEMENT OF PREGNANCY AFTER CESAREAN SECTION

Luis R. Saldana, Harold Schulman, and Lynn Reuss
American Journal of Obstetrics and Gynecology
135 (5):555–561, Nov. 1, 1979

This study was conducted at the Bronx Municipal Hospital Center by the Albert Einstein College of Medicine from 1974 to 1977. A total of 226 women with a low transverse uterine scar were considered for a trial of labor. Of these women, 145 had a trial of labor. The criteria used in their selection were (1) their prenatal care was provided at the special obstetric clinic for high risk mothers, (2) they were known to have had transverse low cervical incisions, and (3) the current pregnancy had been free of complications. Thirty-eight of the women had two or more prior cesareans.

The women were told how to recognize labor and to report to the hospital in early labor. The hospital has twenty-four-hour blood banking (the capacity to prepare blood for transfusions) and the cesarean delivery area was constantly available with adequate anesthesia coverage in the event a cesarean became necessary.

Of the laboring group, 38.6 percent experienced vaginal deliveries. The primary reasons for repeat cesareans in the trial labor group were arrest of active labor and fetal distress. There was no uterine rupture, nor death of mother or child. For the women who tried labor but required a cesarean, 18 percent developed a fever postoperatively. Only 1 percent of the women who experienced vaginal deliveries developed a fever. Of the women who had a repeat scheduled cesarean, 10 percent developed fever postoperatively.

Table 1. Outcome of 145 mothers allowed a trial of labor according to indication for primary cesarean birth.

Indication	Vaginal Delivery Rate
CPD	28%
Fetal Distress	65%
Arrest of Labor	75%
Hypertension	—
Uncertain	43%
Placenta Previa	60%
Breech	—
Failed Induction of Labor	—

The authors of this study conclude: (1) by waiting for labor, maximum fetal growth and lung maturity are assured without the cost of ultrasound and amniocentesis; and (2) their approach (await labor, allow a trial of labor, have available an operating room, anesthesia, and a blood bank) for the otherwise normal mother and infant in the presence of a previous low transverse cesarean scar is safe for both mother and infant.

The two basic safety issues are maternal and fetal death. "Review of the literature and our own results indicate that maternal death is not an issue. Both the probability of gross rupture of the transverse uterine scar and the maternal consequences from it seem largely exaggerated." Strict adherence to a normal labor curve and watchful fetal monitoring is critical for early recognition of distress and early surgical intervention. "There does not seem to be any rational or scientific basis for a 99 percent repeat cesarean section rate in the United States and most well-equipped centers in the United States should abandon this practice."[1]

ABSTRACT: PLANNED VAGINAL DELIVERY FOLLOWING CESAREAN SECTION

Berkeley Merrill and C. E. Gibbs
Obstetrics and Gynecology
52(1):50–52, July 1978

This study was conducted by the University of Texas from 1970 to 1975 (actually the study is continuing but the results are from this five-year period). A total of 526 women with one prior cesarean with a low cervical transverse incision were allowed a trial labor. The patients considered for a trial of labor had (1) a single low cervical incision, and (2) no contraindication to labor and delivery in the current pregnancy (such as transverse, brow, or unfavorable breech presentation, urgent medical indication for delivery such as diabetes, toxemia, placenta previa, and severe pelvic contraction). Of the women who labored, 49 percent delivered vaginally, doing so with a slightly less morbidity (complications) and a shorter hospital stay than 108 similar women not given a trial labor.

All cesareans were done in the labor and delivery suite where a staff physician and an anesthetist were immediately present. The trial of labor was conducted by a staff physician with blood typed and matched and under conditions of careful personal and electronic monitoring of the mother and fetus. Oxytocin was used to induce labor only for premature rupture of the membranes and to augment poor labor contractions in cases of dystocia (abnormal labor). The labor trial continued until vaginal delivery or indication for cesarean occurred. The uterine scar was palpatated manually through the cervix after each vaginal delivery.

The most common reason for the cesarean in the laboring woman was arrest of progress (dilation of cervix and/or descent of baby into birth canal not progressing) or fetal distress. Perinatal (period shortly before and after birth) mortality and morbidity were unaffected by trial of labor or route of delivery. The authors report uterine rupture was encountered three times in the trial group and once in the non-trial group but "at no time resulted in a serious threat to the mother or child."[2] The frequency of uterine rupture was similar to that reported in other studies, i.e., 0.5 percent. "The complication was not serious, with hemorrhage and shock being absent and only one hysterectomy being performed."[3] Noteworthy was the significant increase in complications to the mother found among women whose trial labor resulted in a repeat cesarean as compared to the women who had no labor trial. This difference is especially true in terms of fever, wound complications and blood transfusions. Maternal complications are compared in the table below:

| | Trial of labor | | |
	Vaginal delivery	Abdominal delivery	Abdominal delivery without trial
Maternal mortality	0%	0%	0%
Ruptured uterus	0.6% (2)	0.5% (1)	1% (1)
Anesthesia accident	0%	0%	0%
Blood transfusion	4%	15%	8%
Standard morbidity	5%	38%	9%
Endometritis	4%	26%	7%
Pyelonephritis	3%	9%	2%
Respiratory complications	0.3%	3%	0%
Septicemia	0%	0%	2%
Thromboembolic disorders	0%	0%	1%
Abdominal wound complication	0%	8%	0%
Peritonitis	0.6%	0%	0%

The authors conclude: "We have confirmed what others have found, namely, that approximately half the patients with a previous single low cervical transverse cesarean section can delivery vaginally. We have also confirmed the relative safety of the procedure when conducted in an environment in which the trial can be terminated and abdominal delivery carried out immediately."[4]

Index